# INSIDE/OUTSIDE

# INSIDE/OUTSIDE

*A Physician's Journey
with Cancer*

*by Janet R. Gilsdorf, M.D.*

THE UNIVERSITY OF MICHIGAN PRESS
*Ann Arbor*

2009   2008   2007   2006        4   3   2   1

*A CIP catalog record for this book is available from the British Library.*

Library of Congress Cataloging-in-Publication Data

Gilsdorf, Janet R.
    Inside/outside : a physician's journey with cancer / by Janet R.
Gilsdorf.
        p. cm. — (Conversations in medicine and society)
        Includes bibliographical references and index.
        ISBN-13: 978-0-472-11579-2 (cloth : alk. paper)
        ISBN-10: 0-472-11579-0 (cloth : alk. paper)
        1. Gilsdorf, Janet R.—Health.   2. Breast—Cancer—
Patients—United States—Biography.   3. Pediatricians—United
States—Biography.   4. Physicians—United States—Biography.
I. Title.   II. Series.
RC280.B8G48      2006
362.196'994490092—dc22                          2006008015

*for Jim, Dan, and Joe*

*Foreword*

*The Merriam-Webster Dictionary* defines a journey as the "act or instance of traveling from one place to another." In this eloquent and moving memoir, Dr. Janet Gilsdorf takes the reader on a sometimes painful, and always enlightening journey that captures the complexity of her experience as a breast cancer patient and a physician with a thriving clinic and research laboratory. The book's title, *Inside/Outside,* cogently captures the duality of Dr. Gilsdorf's position on the two—not always cooperative—sides of medical diagnosis and treatment. Moreover, it demonstrates the difficulty of reconciling the two faces of physician and patients once she is cancer-free and returns, on new terms, to a life many blithely and unthinkingly dismiss as "normal."

The charge of our series, Conversations in Medicine and Society, is to deliver accessible and engaging books related to the history and sociology of medicine, health policy, and patient experiences for active readers who care about these subjects. We are delighted to include *Inside/Outside* as the first memoir in the series. It is a captivating narrative exploration of the physical and mental devastation that can ensue after a diagnosis of that disease known generically as "cancer." Fortunately for her readers, patients, and students, Dr. Gilsdorf is so successful at telling her harrowing and life-affirming story as she recounts such events as an awkward breast biopsy, post-chemotherapeutic delirium, and grieving the loss of a full mane of hair. Cancer patients, survivors, and physicians alike will appreciate her candor and rich description of places and characters. We have much to learn from Professor Gilsdorf and her beautifully written book.

In recent years, memoirs have become increasingly popular in American society; in particular, memoirs that poignantly describe individual experiences of physical and mental trauma, pain, and healing.

Sometimes such memoirs veer toward formulaic stories of heroic triumph over adversity and redemption through the suffering of illness. Yet this memoir avoids such a simple narrative progression, as Dr. Gilsdorf's insider medical knowledge complicates her approaches to diagnosis, treatment, and prognosis. As you will soon discover, *Inside/Outside* required a deep courage of expression and self-reflection that is unusual and illuminating.

Using her finely-honed skills as a physician trained to carefully observe and determine the intricacies of a particularly difficult patient case history, Dr. Gilsdorf now casts her gaze inward to the disease that is raging inside her body and the world surrounding those life-altering events. Her gifts of language, communication, and compassion shine on every sentence of this book. Her astute observations on the experience of illness, its conflict with being a physician, and the vague boundaries that divide the world of the well from the world of the ill are nothing short of remarkable and inspiring.

We are fortunate to have Dr. Gilsdorf as a faculty member at the University of Michigan Medical School, a proximity that allowed us to meet frequently during the writing and production process. These intense intellectual and emotional meetings reconfirmed what a marvelous colleague and person she is. As you now peruse and benefit from the wisdom expressed in the pages you are about to turn, we are certain that you will agree.

*Alexandra Minna Stern, Ph.D.*
*Howard Markel, M.D., Ph.D.*

## Author's Note

*This book describes my journey with cancer.* The treatment and medical care I received were appropriate for me at the time it occurred but may not be appropriate for another patient with breast cancer at another time in the evolution of medical therapies.

The identities of my physicians remain obscure so they may continue their important work outside the spotlight's cruel glare. Similarly, the identities of my patients are sacred and hidden. My friends and relatives, on the other hand, are who they are.

For their unending encouragement, I am deeply indebted to my medical and scientific colleagues; to Emmy Holman, Margaret Nesse, Jane Johnson, and Marty Calvert, who read every word several times; to Howard Markel and Alexandra Stern, who got this project started; and to Dr. N., who was always there.

# Contents

# ONE / The Diagnosis

# CHAPTER 1

*"Physician, heal thyself"*

— HIPPOCRATES —

*Today is Valentine's Day,* a day for chocolate hearts and lacy greeting cards, and it begins like every other Monday. I hang my coat on the hook behind my office door and check my calendar: a search committee meeting and a medical education meeting, an interview with a new faculty candidate, a lecture to pediatric residents. In addition, I need to dictate a recommendation letter for a graduate student, return patient phone calls that will accumulate over the next ten hours, revise a scientific paper, and review the lab results from last week's clinic patients. Tony (the three-year-old with septic arthritis): has his sed rate normalized yet? Anna (the sixteen-year-old with a heart transplant and presumed aspergillus in a pulmonary nodule): has her lung tissue grown any fungi yet? Megan (the four-year-old with AIDS): has her CD4 (lymphocytes) count increased or her viral load decreased since we changed her medicines? Today promises to be ordinary, to be filled with the usual.

Tucked into the middle of the morning is an appointment for my annual Pap smear. Irritating and repetitive, it's another of those maintenance duties, as mundane as ordering water softener salt or replacing the furnace filter, as routine as dental checkups, oil changes, and mammograms. I always schedule my annual gyn appointment near my birthday, which is three days after Valentine's Day, so I don't forget.

I was tempted to skip the examination this year but want to talk with my gynecologist about hormone replacement therapy (HRT). I've been taking estrogen and a progesterone for several years because without them I couldn't sleep. Each night I'd awaken at two o'clock, wide-eyed, hot as hell, and drenched in sweat. Rather than falling asleep again, I'd review—forward, backward, and inside out—the work-related dilemmas that paraded relentlessly, trunk-to-tail like circus elephants, through my mind.

I don't like taking medicine for hot flashes. These biologic surges reflect, after all, a normal physiologic transition rather than an illness. Medicines are poisons; they work by fouling up one metabolic pathway or another. Furthermore, HRT is akin to patching an old coat, never as good as the original and sometimes worse than what you started with. My motto over the years had been that nature's way is best, most of the time. But when Mother Nature handed me an unending string of sleepless nights, I was willing to compromise my principles and give her some help.

After I accepted the estrogen-progesterone combination offered by my gynecologist, sleep returned to my nights and enthusiasm to my days. But now I want to ask my doctor if I should stay on the HRTs. Recent studies suggest that estrogens may increase the risk of breast cancer, and they don't seem to protect against heart disease as once thought. Maybe I can do without them. Maybe the hot flashes of old have disappeared.

At the appointment my gynecologist asks the standard, nagging questions about smoking (never), seat belts (always), alcohol (an occasional glass of wine with dinner), supplemental calcium (too hard on the GI tract). Then she examines me. We chat about medical school business—her department, my department—as she palpates my neck, listens to my lungs and heart, prods my abdomen, and slides her fingers over my chest.

She pauses over my left breast, moves to my right breast, and then returns to my left breast. She dwells on the left breast.

"I don't remember this lump from before," she says.

She asks me to feel it. I run my index and middle fingers over the surface of my left breast and push against the soft tissue. It feels normal, like fine-grained bubble wrap. My fingers move an inch. Normal. They move another inch. There it is. Above and medial to my left nipple. A firm almond.

"Have you felt that before?" she asks.

"No." I explain that several years ago, following a minor breast lump scare, I vowed that every Sunday while in the shower I would shave my legs and perform a breast self-examination. And every Sunday since, I have shaved my legs and have not examined my breasts. Why not? I don't know, other than the obvious: if I don't look, I won't find.

"I can't tell if it's another cyst in your otherwise cystic breasts or something to be more concerned about," she says.

"My husband's a general surgeon, you know." Actually, she probably doesn't know this detail about me. "I'll have him check it." Jim takes care of many women with breast masses; some need biopsies, some need fine needle aspirates, many need reassurance. He'll clear this up. He'll dispel any question of the lump being worrisome. He'll recognize it as a cyst.

It's late when I get home from work, and Jim arrives even later. We read the newspapers and the mail and stir-fry pork and vegetables for our Valentine's Day supper. He pays the mortgage and electricity bills. I knit two more inches on the sweater I'm making for my daughter-in-law. The lump doesn't cross my mind.

The next night, Tuesday, I attend a dinner for a visiting professor. Then, at home, I undress and slip into bed, again forgetting about the lump.

Wednesday night I go to a Murray Perahia piano recital. For years my friend Sally and I have had season tickets to the Choral Union Concert Series. Neither of our husbands can take that much good music, so we go together.

After the concert, I hang my jacket in the closet, pull off my sweater, step out of my skirt, and shed my underwear. Maybe it's the cool air against my bare chest that makes me remember. Maybe it's the weight of a concern I have refused to acknowledge. As I squirm into my nightgown, I say to my husband, "Oh, by the way, my gynecologist found a lump in my breast." To give him the right context, I add, "I'm sure it's a cyst."

"Hop up on the bed," he says. "Let me take a look."

I pull off the nightgown and lie down. Staring at the top of the bed board, he kneads my breasts and digs his fingertips into my armpits. Like my gynecologist, he moves from the left breast to the right and then returns to the left. He dwells on my left breast.

Straightening up, he steps back. The light from the bedside lamp shines off his thick white hair like twilight off a pearl. His face is somber and professional. His eyes, usually sparkling, are now dull. This is the doctor his patients see. He folds his arms across his chest and quietly says, "If you were in my office, I'd put a needle in it."

He's being cautious, as he is in his surgical practice. How many times has he said that fear of litigation drives many surgeons to biopsy masses they know aren't malignant? In the United States, he says, about eighteen biopsies are done for every breast cancer found. I know this lump is just an ordinary cyst, and I don't want to be bothered with a procedure. I have too many things to do, including a trip to visit our son who is in the navy and stationed in Monterey, California. We're scheduled to leave Friday, the day after tomorrow.

"I'll take care of it after we get back from the West Coast." I put my nightgown back on. "A couple days won't make any difference."

He agrees that the fine needle aspirate can wait. His opinion on this is more authoritative than mine, for breast lumps and cancers and cysts and biopsies and mastectomies are his professional bread and butter, while I deal with serious infections in children, those that are difficult to diagnose, difficult to treat. Following our return from California, I figure, he can aspirate the lump one evening in his office. That way I won't have to deal with making an appointment at the University Health System, won't have to spend hours in the surgery clinic, won't have to lose a day at work. The lump is, after all, just a cyst.

On Thursday Jim cooks a birthday dinner for me, guided by a recipe from D'ARTAGNAN's *Glorious Game Cookbook*, one of his favorites. He has defrosted a pheasant and, after sprinkling salt and pepper into its cavity, adds a dollop of mustard. Then he jams a large onion into the bird and ties its legs with a piece of string. Jim enjoys cooking odd things, and while the bird simmers in the oven, he makes a salad of lettuce, dill pickles, and blue cheese. To go with the pheasant, he braises cabbage and concocts a sauce of meat drippings, cream, and bourbon. With a wooden spoon in one hand and a glass of Jack

Daniels in the other, he stirs the sauce and sips the booze. His eyes glisten with delight, and he hums the title song from *Paint Your Wagon*.

It's a magical evening: good food, good wine, my fondest companion. Outside, beyond the dining room window, the glare of moonlight off the snow outlines the twisted limbs of the cherry tree. Inside, the warm, flickering glow from the candles spreads like honey over the table.

When we finish eating, I mention the breast lump aspirate again. "What kind of painkiller do you use?"

"None."

"NONE?!?!" I'm amazed. "You stick a big old needle into someone's breast without local anesthesia?"

"It's a thin needle."

"That's cruel."

"No, it isn't. The pain from infiltrating the skin with Lidocaine is worse than the needle poke."

"How about EMLA (topical anesthetic)?" I suggest. "Works great for spinal taps on kids."

"Never heard of it. Sounds like overkill to me."

"Well," I take a deep, impatient breath, "let me educate you."

I pull the *Physician's Desk Reference*, the often-consulted "PDR," from the bookshelf and read aloud about EMLA.

"I'm not convinced," he says, yawning. This is his silent way of saying that he doesn't like the conversation. "It really isn't that bad."

"You don't own a breast." I make a mental note to write myself a prescription for EMLA so I can smear it over the lump an hour before he needles it.

This is our first visit to the Monterey Peninsula, and, starting with a snowstorm before leaving Michigan, it hasn't gone well. Ours is the last plane to leave, albeit late, before Detroit Metro Airport is shut down.

We land in San Jose late in the afternoon, rent a car, and drive Route 17 west through the canyons of the Santa Cruz Mountains.

Clogged with evening rush hour traffic, the road is a snake of bumper-to-bumper cars whirling around the curves at sixty miles per hour. The California State Highway Department is improving the intersection with Highway 1, so we idle in gridlock for about an hour. After two wrong turns into Monterey, tired and frustrated, we finally locate our hotel, a turn-of-the-century downtown classic, with high ceilings and no on-site parking. The historic elevator, which seemed charming from the Web site description, is on the fritz, so we haul our luggage up the stairs to the third floor. Our room, fortunately, is tastefully decorated and comfortable. Best of all, from its huge window we glimpse a wedge of Monterey Bay twinkling in the sun three blocks away.

Several years ago, Joe, our younger son, traveled around the world on the USS *Samuel Gompers*, where he was responsible for the bow anchor. He completed his military obligation, discovered again that college was not for him, and reenlisted. Now he has just begun a tour of duty at the Defense Language Institute at the Presidio of Monterey, where he will learn French. Since graduating from high school, he has been in an independent phase, so we haven't seen or heard from him much. He doesn't have a telephone in his room—too cheap to pay for one—and doesn't have a cell phone—ditto—so we have been dependent on his rare calls home from a pay phone.

Jim and I wait for Joe in the Crown and Anchor Bar. We haven't seen our son in months. Will he still have his closely clipped military haircut? Will he have gained, or lost, weight? Will he still have his contrary attitude? Every time the door opens, a streak of light blazes into the dark tavern, and I turn expectantly toward the person entering. Will Joe be sullen or chatty or distant? He's capable of any of these moods. Finally the door opens, a bright flash slices across our table, and Joe ambles in.

"Howdy," he calls.

He's beautiful, with his enlistment hairdo, with thrust-back shoulders that tell of pride. I dash over to him and wrap my arms around his neck. His stiff muscles tell me he's embarrassed.

Drinking British beer and eating shepherd's pie, we listen to Joe's navy stories. His laughing baritone assures me that he has finally figured out how to have fun. The elaborately detailed accounts of golf matches, dart tournaments, and snooker (a game I've never heard of) remind me that he's an adult now and I must let go of the little boy I worried over so much.

Besides overlooking a sliver of Monterey Bay, the huge window in our hotel room, unfortunately, also overlooks Alvarado Street. Car after car loaded with screaming teenagers spews thumping music and trolls the road immediately below us. It's three o'clock in the morning (six o'clock Michigan time), and I haven't slept at all. Disconnected thoughts stream like an endless newsreel through my mind. I think about the flight, this evening with Joe in the British bar, our upcoming visit to the Monterey Bay Aquarium.

I roll over in bed, nudging Jim with my foot, and hope that Joe will find his place in linguistics, in the navy, in the world. The newsreel continues to spool. I think about being fifty-five years old, about the way 1999 lurched into 2000 six weeks ago, about the progress of the new millennium. I think about the children of the world and about their parents, doing, for the most part, the best they can.

Thoughts of the lump swing back into my mind again. I imagine myself in Jim's office, lying on the examining table, EMLA cream smeared over the lump. I see him poised over my chest with a needle. I see him dispassionately jabbing it into my breast.

My fingers stroke the firm almond nestled in the tissues above my left nipple. It's still there. I pull my hand back, thinking that if it *is* cancer and I massage it too hard or too often, I might force a shower of malignant cells into my bloodstream, and they could lodge in distant places and grow into metastases. Of course, the lump in my breast *isn't* cancer, but my hand stays riveted to the bed sheet anyway.

Disturbed by the racket in the street below, I roll over yet again and consider the amazing ability of the human mind to perform leaping gymnastics when it ought to be resting.

What if this isn't a cyst? What if it's really cancer? I think of Natalie, a woman I never met. Years ago I read her story in the newspaper. It's the foundation for the cancer illusion I have carried ever since. Natalie was a pediatrician, like me, and she had breast cancer. Her friends arranged for someone to accompany her to every chemotherapy session and then stay with her for several days. Ultimately, she died; the newspaper story was her obituary. In my cancer illusion, alone and green with nausea, I'm driving the freeway home from my chemo infusion and balancing a mixing bowl, half full of vomit, in my lap. Even though I have absolutely no risk factors and no family history of a malignancy, ever since reading about Natalie I've known deep in my bones I'm doomed to cancer. Maybe this is a leftover from the helplessness of childhood. Maybe I'm haunted by a deep-seated but unknown fear from long ago. Growing up in North Dakota, I learned to fear freezing to death, to fear getting lost and starving to death, to fear drowning in the Red River, but I don't remember fearing cancer. Wherever it came from, I'm convinced that a tumor is my fate and that I will have to face it alone. Sick and alone. Eventually. But not now. This is a cyst.

On our last day in Monterey, the carefully planned visit to the aquarium isn't going well either. Joe is two hours late. Since he has no phone, we can't call him. Early this morning, responding to our internal clocks that are stuck in the eastern time zone, Jim and I awoke at six o'clock.

I wait for Joe in the hotel lobby and read *Cannery Row* for the second time. John Steinbeck wrote, or at least conceived, the book here in this town. As I breathe the mist off the bay that he breathed, watch the waves rush past the rocks that he watched, hear the screams of the seagulls that he heard, the book and its kooky characters come to life. Cannery Row, the street, is now a tourist trap. In Steinbeck's day it was filthy, noisy, smelly, and ironically named Ocean View. Its view, then, of the Pacific was blocked by hulking canneries. Still, I'm enchanted with the story and the place and the people.

Three hours overdue, Joe saunters through the hotel's front door. "Hi," he calls and offers no explanation for his tardiness. I don't want to ruin the end of our visit, so I keep the about-to-detonate anger bomb locked deep in my explosion-proof internal vault.

The aquarium is about a mile from the hotel, and I want to drive. Jim and Joe want to walk, so we walk. The trail along the bay is littered with sightseers, but I hardly notice them. Rather, I look beyond the crowd to the marina, to the languid seals on the rocks, to the roiling waves. I don't feel well. Nothing specific, just a little throb behind my eyes, a few vague aches, and a general sense of being out of whack.

It's a three-day weekend and hundreds of visitors swarm into the aquarium. Watching the slow dance of the kelp as it turns and sways in its three-story tank makes me woozy. In the ladies' room I splash water over my face and rest awhile. I'm never sick, so what's this all about? Probably exhaustion from not sleeping.

Saying good-bye to Joe as we leave Monterey is difficult. I want more of his hearty laugh, of his crazy navy stories. He's the kid who, even as a baby, refused to dance with me, who wouldn't release his body to any kind of twist or rhythm. But he's growing up. His arms and legs reel in jerky contortions as he punctuates his navy tales with the navy walk. Although he may not recognize it, the military has been very good for him. It offers the structure and predictability he needs to find his way. I give him a farewell hug, and he pats my shoulder.

On the drive back to the San Jose airport, this time on Highway 101 to avoid the canyons in the Santa Cruz Mountains, we pass through Gilroy, the "Garlic Capitol of the World." Even though the car windows are shut, the pungent essence in the air finds its way inside. For some odd reason, while surrounded by garlic I'm thinking about doctors. About Jim's three brothers who are all surgeons. About surgical procedures. About the stringent smell of disinfectant that permeates all things medical. About the Saturday night in Alaska when our older son, Daniel, then two years old, cut open his eyebrow.

In violation of the household rules, Daniel was using our bed as a trampoline. With a misstep on a bounce he crash-landed and slammed his eyebrow against the corner of the dresser. The cut was about an inch long and bled like a fountain. We clapped a washrag over the wound and headed across the parking lot from our apartment to the Indian Health Service hospital, where Jim was stationed as a U.S. Public Health Service physician.

Daniel lay on the emergency room table wrapped like a papoose in a draw sheet. While I held our squirming son down, Jim sewed his eyebrow up. In the middle of the screaming, Daniel's wide, wild eyes—flooded with tears—skewered mine as if to say, "Why are you doing this to me? You're my parents! You're supposed to protect me." I vowed we would never again be his doctors.

Yet, a few years later, Daniel returned from a week at Boy Scout camp with a low-grade fever, a sore throat, and a voice that sounded as if a gym sock were stuffed in his mouth. I examined his pharynx, using a dinner knife as a tongue depressor, and discovered suspicious swelling of his palate and a very groady-looking right tonsil. In spite of my earlier vow, I gave him sample antibiotics from the bathroom drawer. He did fine. But this was probably an early peritonsillar abscess, and treating it myself was a dumb thing to do.

A wise, old, but still valid rule of medicine cautions a physician against treating herself or friends or family members. As is said about lawyers, a physician who treats himself has a fool for a doctor. Objective decision making (and medical decisions are *best* made objectively) requires the physician-patient relationship to be unencumbered by passion or sentiment or intimate familiarity. In rendering clinical judgments, we physicians acquire our information—data from the medical history and physical examination and laboratory test results—at a prescribed distance. Shorten the measuring stick, move the target closer, and the stakes go up; we process the information differently and, in all likelihood, less accurately.

After the long flight back to Michigan from California, Jim and I sit in our family room, me in my favorite easy chair and him resting his sore back in the La-Z-Boy recliner, and talk again about the fine needle aspirate. Tonight I see this procedure differently than before our trip out west. Maybe it's because of the waters of Monterey Bay that crash against the rocks and send sparkling spindrift high into the air. Maybe it's because Joe seems comfortable in his new place. Maybe it's because I remembered the rule about doctors and their families. My decision to have Jim do the fine needle aspirate begins to waver.

I'm certain Jim doesn't want to be my doctor, and yet he knows more about breast disease, including cancer, than many of the other surgeons in this community. I don't want him to be my doctor, yet I trust him more than any other person on the planet.

"Jim," I say, stroking the almond in my left breast for the thousandth time, "what if it's positive?"

His silence fills the room. The furnace fan whirs. Warm air blows through the house, stirring the leaves on the ficus plant.

"If the path report comes back positive," I say, "you'll have to tell me."

"That's right." His hushed words sound like a prayer.

I pause for a long minute. "That would be awful, honey; awful for you and awful for me."

He nods.

"I'll call another surgeon," I say. "Tomorrow. Someone at the university. Name one."

*"Physician, heal thyself"*

# CHAPTER 2

*Egalitarianism Bumps against Personal Needs*

*During the many years I have practiced medicine*, I, a tireless advocate of basic health care for every American, have always taken the high road. To me, all young people have equal value and every ill child deserves the best care that pediatrics can offer. Contrary to the adult world, in the world of children, there are no "executive health plans" for "corporate" kids.

Yet reality reigns. Ordinary patients cannot pick up the phone, dial the office of a senior surgeon at the University Cancer Center, and immediately connect with him. That's exactly what I do on the Monday morning after returning from California.

"Dr. Gleason's office." His secretary, the person responsible for shielding him against phone calls, answers.

"This is Dr. Gilsdorf from Pediatric Infectious Diseases." I use my stern, rapid-paced doctor voice. "I'm trying to reach Dr. Gleason." I know how to cut through the smoke thrown by a doctor's office staff. This approach has worked a million times when I've needed to reach a colleague on behalf of a patient.

"Let me check, Dr. Gilsdorf." She pauses a moment and then says, "Yes, he's off the phone now. I'll put you right through."

Several electronic clicks later, Myron answers. "Janet, what can I do for you?"

I know him from hospital committees, from medical school memos. He is, however, not my doctor, as I've never had a health problem that requires an operation. Furthermore, since he's a cancer surgeon who cares for adult patients and I'm a pediatric infectious diseases specialist, we've never even taken care of a patient together. He has the right distance to be a good physician for me.

"Well, Myron, last week Susan Fridley—she's my gynecologist—found a lump in my left breast. Jim thinks it needs to be biopsied."

Myron and Jim have worked together in the past, and Jim has considerable respect for Myron's sensible approach to surgical problems, for his efficiency during operations, for his "good hands" and "good head." Since Jim isn't doing the procedure himself, I want him to be comfortable with my surgeon. Until now, I've always made decisions about my health with no input from my husband. This time I let him choose my doctor.

"Okay, Janet. I can see you in my clinic tomorrow morning. We'll get a mammogram first. Go to radiology in the Cancer Center about 10:00, and then I'll see you at 12:30. I'll set up the appointment and get a requisition to the x-ray department. Do you have your hospital registration number handy?"

It's as simple as that. If I were a normal patient, setting up this consultation would have been very different. I would have called the Cancer Center appointment line, would have been put on hold and told by an electronic operator that I'm number three . . . or five . . . or worse . . . in queue. I would have spent ten minutes listening to an automated woman with a flight attendant voice promote the University Health System. When a human finally got on the line, I would have been given an appointment for several weeks later with whichever doctor was available that day.

I'm a bit embarrassed that my egalitarianism has gone right out the window, for calling Myron directly seems a little like cheating. Yet, I'm a long-term member of the "physician family" at this medical center. In spite of my high-road ideals about health-care equality, this time I want to cut through the bureaucratic clutter and get the job done quickly.

Small clusters of people, each containing a patient and at least one support person, dot the radiology reception area in the Cancer Center.

Alone, I take a seat beside the aquarium and watch the fish. Elegant in their scaly coats of metallic blue, green, and lilac, they swim without a care among the weeds. Snails, one drab brown and another muddy gray, slide along the sandy bottom on pads of slime and vacuum up the waste.

At this moment, my husband is "scrubbed." He's in the operating room of the hospital across town, taking care of someone else's spouse. I don't bitterly ask myself why he isn't here. I know. The stabs of loneliness that stir my insides are countered by my understanding that the patient comes first. Doesn't matter if it's a weekend, the middle of the night, or a terribly inconvenient moment. Doesn't matter if the patient is rich or poor, a saint or a criminal, charming or a pain in the ass. The supremacy of the patient's needs is, after all, the essence of the Hippocratic Oath—our promise to treat the sick to the best of our ability, to preserve patient privacy, to recognize and value the humanity of those we serve, to teach the art and science of medicine to the next generation, to recognize our own limitations. Rather than pull us apart, this pledge that Jim and I each took years ago is embraced and honored by us both.

Last night we discussed whether he should accompany me to the appointment with Myron.

"My schedule is chock-full," Jim said, leafing through his pocket calendar.

"That's okay," I said, really meaning it. I imagined the people he will operate on today. Maybe an old woman will have her gallbladder removed and her three sons have traveled a total of fifteen hundred miles to be with her. Maybe a businessman will have his colon cancer resected and has rearranged his work schedule to accommodate the six-week recovery time.

"It's only a crummy little cyst, definitely not worth destroying the OR schedule for an entire day," I said. "You'll get a full report from me tomorrow night."

This morning, on his way out the back door, Jim wrapped his arms around me and said, "I wish I could be there with you."

Mammograms are torture. Mammograms afford no dignity. Naked from the waist up, I stand at the x-ray machine, my bare breast clamped between two cold metal plates. As the old joke about mammograms goes: first you take two dictionaries out of the freezer; second, you place your breast between them; third, you lie down in the driveway and have your husband drive his truck back and forth over the books.

Back in the radiology waiting room, with my hospital gown on backwards to afford easy access to my chest, I'm waiting to be told that it's okay to get dressed, waiting for the radiologist to scan the films for quality. If they're not optimal, the technician will have to retake them.

I dislike the waiting room, dislike the babble and laugh tracts from the television, dislike the plastic-covered furniture. The presence of the other patients irritates me. They are curious about my health. I don't want to talk to them, don't want to hear about their problems. If I could wait alone in a little cubicle, behind a wall, behind a curtain, I'd be happier. But I can't. I hide behind my medical journal, unable to concentrate on what I'm reading because of the television noise and the comings and goings of the other patients.

"Dr. Gilsdorf?" The technician who calls my name is tall and blond, and her theatrical smile reminds me of Delores Bell, my mother's friend during my childhood. Delores was the only divorced woman I knew while I was growing up. To my young eyes, she was tainted in some way, very suspect, yet she was very enigmatic, very intriguing.

"The radiologist would like to speak with you."

This has happened before. During previous mammograms, the radiologist has told me the final reading before I left the x-ray suite. I'm not sure this is standard procedure. It may be reserved for members of the "physician family."

As we walk down the hallway, the technician slides her arm around my shoulders. My back stiffens. Her touch is too familiar, is as irritating as if she had called me "honey" or "dear." The old system of medical hierarchy makes its stand. She's a technician whom I have never met and I'm a physician. Above all, it's very odd.

The radiologist is also a stranger. In the shadows of the darkened reading room, she sits before a row of view boxes, their back-lit panels covered with black, white, and gray x-ray films. She introduces herself, a Greek name consistent with both the tangle of black curls that spread over her shoulders and the melodic, softly foreign accent of her voice.

She stares deep into my eyes and says, haltingly, "We see the lump that you feel, but not very well. It shows up best on only one view. I want to be sure you have contacted a surgeon."

A deep dread begins to slink into my awareness, clawing its way forward like an ominous reptile, creeping to the edge of my knowing. I send it scurrying back with the admonition, *this is just a cyst.* "I have an appointment with Myron Gleason this afternoon."

As I pull on my clothes in the dressing room, I consider the three eerie things: the technician's arm around my shoulder; the cryptic words of the radiologist; and Jim's immediate certainty that the lump needed to be biopsied. The deep dread raises its gruesome head again. Maybe this isn't as simple as a cyst. The radiologist must have seen something suspicious in that mammogram film. Well, I remind myself, cysts can be suspicious.

A half hour later, undressed again from the waist up, I'm sitting on an examining table in the surgical oncology clinic of the Cancer Center. The door flies open and Myron swoops in, coat tails aflutter. In any medical encounter, the doctor's entrance—the arrival of the healer— is a powerful thing. Suddenly, as electric as lightning, confidence charges the room where worry once prevailed. Upon the appearance of the physician, something will happen. A decision. An opinion. Action of some sort.

"Hello, Janet. Good to see you."

Yes, I think, I wish the circumstances were different.

He stares at my chest, looking for asymmetry of my nipples. He examines my breasts, first the left, then the right, then the left again. He feels for nodes in my armpit. With a sigh, he steps back, purses his lips, and nods. Then he says, "Well, I certainly agree with Jim. This needs to be needled. It's all set up for the pathologist to do it today."

We physicians are very bad at ministering to ourselves and to the people we love. Here I lie, on an examining table in the bowels of the Cancer Center, about to have a fine needle aspirate of my breast, and my husband is elsewhere.

In some ways, I'm glad to be alone. At least this way, I don't have to take care of him during this visit, don't have to answer his questions, don't have to justify the way fine needle aspirates are done in the University Health System. I've never learned to let him comfort me in situations like this. In truth, he's usually not very good at comfort. If he were here, he would protect his own feelings and maintain the same distance from me as from his patients. That's the only way he knows how to deal with sick people.

When I was pregnant with Daniel, our first child, Jim kept saying he didn't want to be in the delivery room, didn't want to watch the obstetrician deliver the baby, didn't want to be around if something went wrong. I told him the doctor's job was to handle the business at my bottom and the husband's job was to handle the business at my head, to help me get through it.

Indeed, while I was in labor—in the middle of the night, in the dead of winter, at the end of the earth in the Mountain Home Air Force Base hospital in Idaho—Jim wasn't very useful. Daniel was occiput posterior (face up), and toward the end of a long, grueling labor my obstetrician wanted me to push hard in an attempt to turn the baby's head. So I pushed. And pushed. And pushed. The more I pushed, the whiter Jim's face became.

Finally, he commanded, "Janet, breathe."

A loud groan exploded from me as I exhaled. "Look," I gasped, "I can't push and breathe at the same time. Right now I'm going to push." He upset me so much that I asked him to stay in the waiting room with his mother.

While I was in labor with Joe, our second child, at the Indian Health Service hospital in Bethel, Alaska, Jim spent the entire night in the trauma bay, sewing up the cut hand of an Alaskan fisherman named Oscar Wilbur. My husband was clearly more comfortable in the emergency room with Oscar than in the labor room with me.

Now, fifteen minutes after Myron examined me, I'm in a procedure room. The examining table is covered with crinkly, white paper; fluorescent lights glare overhead; nicked plaster dots the edges of the beige walls. The stainless steel countertop is bare except for a microscope and staining materials, the equipment the pathologist will use to assess the material he will aspirate from my breast.

The door opens and a pot-bellied man with red-orange hair walks in, followed by a younger woman with a slight limp. The man shuffles a stack of papers.

"Left breast, right?" He stares at the papers rather than at me.

I'm not sure who the question is for. I answer anyway. "Yes, the left side." I cross my ankles and adjust my hair, which is trapped between the back of my head and the examining table's paper cover. "Upper, inner quadrant." My fingers caress the lump. It's still there.

Apparently he doesn't hear me. Or else he's ignoring me. He slams the papers on the counter and whirls like a top toward me. Seems as if he's having a bad day. Worse than mine? His hand kneads my left breast. He nods and mumbles to himself, "There it is."

As he runs a swab soaked with cold antiseptic over my breast and wipes away a clear path with a piece of gauze, he explains to the young woman what he's doing. I assume she's a pathology resident—her name tag says "[Something] [Something], M.D., Dep't of Pathology."

"Little stick," he says, dangling a needle attached to a syringe over my breast.

The young woman resident takes my hand and asks, "You okay?"

I nod. "What size needle is that?"

"Twenty-three gauge," the man answers.

Pretty thin, I tell myself. Won't leave a big hole.

"Try to relax," the young woman says. "It's easier when you're relaxed."

The needle rams through my skin. My eyelids clamp shut. *It hurts.* He runs the tip of the needle up and down inside my breast. *This really hurts.*

When I made the appointment for today, I didn't realize they'd do the fine needle aspirate immediately. I expected to be examined and given another appointment for the procedure. While pleased with the efficiency, I'm not exactly prepared. Further, as Jim would have done, this doctor is performing this procedure with no pain relief. I must remember to tell my husband to use EMLA on all his fine needle aspirates.

How much does it hurt? As much as delivering a baby? As much as having an embedded IUD yanked out of my uterus? On a scale of one to ten, is this an eight or a ten or a twelve? Pain scales are a useless academic exercise here. It hurts like hell, and I have to tough it out.

The young resident strokes my forehead. The pathologist pulls the needle from my breast and works on the specimen at the counter.

Wait, I scream to myself. Wait a goddamn minute. Who is this guy? He didn't introduce himself to me. He might be the janitor or the parking lot attendant for all I know, although his name tag also says "[Something] [Something], M.D., Dep't of Pathology." This jerk just jammed a needle into my breast without telling me who he is. Obviously he doesn't know that I'm a physician, didn't bother to learn anything about his patient. Anyway, it doesn't matter that I'm a doctor. No one should be treated like this.

Why is a pathologist performing this procedure, anyway? Everyone knows that medical students become pathologists because they don't want to interact with intact people. They want to deal only with tissues and cells and body fluids.

I'm mad. My breast throbs as if stung by a hornet. My sense of equilibrium is tied in knots. I might be in the process of learning that I have cancer. I'm alone. I'm scared.

Some patients in this ugly situation would be in-your-face aggressive. They would lash out at the pathologist, would try to hurt him as he had hurt them. But besides being mad, I'm also the product of my North Dakota, Scandinavian heritage: passive, go-along-to-get-along, polite, nicer than nice. When my guard is down, these traits—my cultural destiny—bubble to the top, for they are the default settings of my personality.

In my role as physician, I don't do my best work when I'm accused or assaulted or the target of abuse. Right now I need this pathologist to do his best with this biopsy. Even more than knowing who he is, I need him to get a decent sample. So I lie here, wordless, waiting for it to be over, waiting for him to go away.

"Not enough cells," he mutters to himself. Then he jabs the needle into my breast again.

Still not enough cells. He turns to the resident.

"Have you done one of these yet?" he asks her. "Give it a try."

She jams the needle into my lump. The tip slides up and down like a piston inside my breast. I sense the faintest scritch scritch tucked between the throbs of pain. I try to listen, to hear it more clearly, but it isn't a sound. It's a sensation. It feels gritty, like sticking a dressmaker's pin into my sand-filled pin cushion.

A parade of stereotypes fills this room, led by the male pathologist and the female resident. He is the senior. She is the junior. He is the supervisor. She is the trainee. He is gruff. She tries to be gentle. They are the doctors. I am the patient.

The pathologist mutters to himself as he stares into the microscope. The resident strokes my forehead again. Her touch isn't soothing. I want this fiasco to be over so I can get away from both of them.

The pathologist stomps back to the examining table and picks up yet another needle. "Still not enough cells."

He's exasperated. I'm furious that he's exasperated or, rather, furious that I *know* he's exasperated. I don't care how he feels except that I want this procedure to be done and to be done adequately. I can't say I want it done right. It's too late for that. Already it's been done very wrong. I just want him to get a good sample. A familiar churning clutches my stomach; it happens when I have to watch someone struggle and can't do anything about it.

The pathologist jabs the needle into my breast yet again, the fourth stab, and drives it up and down, scritch scritch, again. Tears puddle in the corners of my eyes and run down my temples into my ears. Have I ever failed to introduce myself to a patient? I surely hope not. Next time I take care of patients, I'll introduce myself twice to be sure I haven't forgotten.

He pulls the needle out of my breast and checks the sample in the microscope.

What's he looking for? Cancer, of course, ultimately. But first he has to be sure that the specimen is of high enough quality. Later, the cells in the sample will be examined in more detail in the pathology laboratory. But first he needs to be sure that he has enough material and that, rather than just fat cells, the sample contains cells from other structures in my breast as well.

"Finally," he sighs. His exasperation seems to have lightened a bit. "It's a good specimen."

Thank God. At this moment the question of cancer is secondary for me. The primary issue is that I no longer have to endure either the needle or these pathologists.

They head out the door.

"What do I do now?" I say to their backs.

"Wait here."

# CHAPTER 3

## The Power of Language

*A half hour after the fine needle aspirate* I'm back in the examining room. Myron sweeps through the door again, this time with less flair. A sense of impending badness taints everything around me like a shadow that grows longer and longer and darker and darker before the relentless fall of the setting sun. I know what he's going to say. All the signs have pointed to it.

"Well, Janet." His voice is soft and solemn. His gaze is direct, drilling into my core. I couldn't stand for him to look away. "The fine needle aspirate shows carcinoma."

Carcinoma. It's a slap, a fierce, stinging bull's-eye. The word reverberates through my brain in massive, coal-colored, high-energy spasms. Carcinoma. Carcinoma. I know exactly what that is; learned it thirty years ago in medical school; have used the word possibly ten thousand times. Until six seconds ago, carcinoma was cancer of the epithelium, of cells that line the internal and external surfaces of our organs. Now, carcinoma is the cancer that is growing inside me.

Myron keeps talking, and I hear only splinters of what he says. His voice weaves and bobs like a water sprite, in and out of the waves that crash through my head: ". . . as you know . . .", ". . . choices . . . ," ". . . lumpectomy with radiation . . . ," ". . . mastectomy . . . ," "axillary dissection . . . ," ". . . sentinel node biopsy . . ." He is far, far away and yet very near. His words pile on top of each other, as off-center as a three-year-old's tower of blocks, and yet, one . . . by . . . one, his words string out a yard apart.

Carcinoma hangs in this examining room like a rotten smell. Its gnarly fingers crawl out of every crevice and eat up every molecule of clean air. It won't go away. It's smothering me.

"Talk with Jim," Myron says. "Take all the time you need. There's no hurry in making these decisions." He pauses, and then the corners of his mouth bow into a brief smile. "But, for your information, I happen to have an open OR slot on Friday."

I smile in return. He completely understands that I won't stew over this, that I'll be decisive. "Jim and I will discuss my options tonight," I manage to say, "and I'll get back to you tomorrow."

Myron leaves. I'm alone in the examining room with my raw, new identity.

Cancer is a heart-stopping word. Its very sound is ominous. The word begins, like a kick, with a harsh, guttural "câ," moves to a whiney "ân," and drops off quickly to a nearly inaudible "sur." Its six short letters carry an uncommonly heavy weight. Written or spoken, the word evokes wrenching terror, elicits images of pain and suffering and dying.

How did this word get attached to me? The pathologist did it. "CANCER" codifies the images he saw. Hunched over the microscope, his eyebrows brushing against the oculars, he stared at the material he had aspirated from my breast lump and studied the clumps of cells, now stained purple, blue, and pink. First, to establish a baseline against which he would decide if abnormal cells were present, he looked for normal breast cells. He searched for milk gland cells and duct cells and fat cells and strands of fibrous stroma, the scaffolding that holds the whole thing together. He recognized the normal cells because they were uniform in shape and size and had the appearance of cells from normal breasts.

Against the background of normal cells he looked for abnormal cells, for clumps of cells that were irregular in shape and size, a mixture of huge cells and tiny cells and everything in between. Normal cells are monotonously the same. Cancer cells are riotously variable. They have larger nuclei, the blue-stained, round command centers of the cells, in relationship to their cytoplasm, the gel-like filler. Their chromatin, strings of DNA in the chromosomes, appears clumped, while nucleoli, the staging site for protein assembly, are present as dark blue dots. The cytoplasm of cancer cells is clear, free of the trash that clogs the cytoplasm of normal cells.

If these cells were just images, they would be beautiful, colorful, varied, rhythmic. As mere images to the casual observer, they would carry no meaning. But for the pathologist, and for me, they carry a great burden of meaning.

As he stared into the microscope, my pathologist needed to attach a name to what he saw. He sat at a fork in the road, and the lane to the left—cancer—leads to a very different place than that to the right—no cancer. He had criteria; he followed guidelines from his professional societies that foster consistency in the application of these names. Clinical studies over the years have correlated the cellular patterns he sees with what happens to the patient. He is experienced and has examined many samples of "cancer" and "not cancer." Yet, this decision may be somewhat arbitrary. When gazing at my specimen, did he correctly place the cells into the right category? Were the cells a little too irregular to proclaim "negative for cancer" or not quite irregular enough to proclaim "positive for cancer"?

The stakes, of course, are high. "Negative" sends the message that all is well. "Positive," on the other hand, sends the doctor and the patient down an entirely different track, a very bumpy road riddled with land mines.

What if he was wrong? What if he called my cells cancer when, indeed, they were normal or the result of a weird inflammatory, nonmalignant process? Then I would be treated with a disfiguring operation, potentially lethal drugs, and high-dose radiation when I didn't need any of it or, worse yet, needed a different kind of therapy. What if he had called my cells normal when, indeed, they were cancer? Then I would miss an opportunity to be treated earlier rather than later.

Biology, however, does not exist as a dichotomy. Rather than black or white, it splays, like a rainbow, along a colorful continuum. Some specimens my pathologist has examined might have been a close call. They may have had a few features of cancer but not all. They may have had features of normal tissue but in some ways resembled cancer. He couldn't waffle. My biopsy had to be either positive or negative. Ambiguous words such as "might be cancer" or "might be normal" couldn't be used. If doubts clouded his certainty, he would have informally consulted with colleagues or sent the tissue to a national expert. If he were still stumped, he would have said the specimen contains cancer cells to avoid the risk of missing one. With this potentially fatal disease, it's better to receive unnecessary treatment than no treatment.

As he stared into his microscope the pathologist spoke into a Dictaphone, transforming the images before him into words. He dumped the characteristics of the cells he visualized into the crucible of his mind, passed these observations through the filters of his training and experience, and then tempered them with his judgment. Finally, he assigned a diagnosis: ductal carcinoma. With those two words, he set me and my doctors on a course of no return.

Alone in the examining room, the heft of cancer is too much for me. Rather than embrace it, I need to avoid it, so I do what I do best, focus on the medical details and leap into action. The immense world of medicine—full of facts, mechanisms, treatment plans, schedules, clinical studies, and expert opinions—offers a comfortable refuge for me. What Myron has just told me flips through my head like pages from a medical textbook.

It's easy for me to listen to the clinical jargon. I love our language of medicine, the way the words, many of them rooted in Latin, ferry ideas, concepts, and details between physicians. There is poetry in these words, *electrocardiograph, dysplasia, type and cross-match, cytology, lymphadenectomy, radionuclide lymphoscintigraphy.*

Right now for me, cancer is a disease process, a mass of cells that I visualize from my memory of slides in my medical school pathology class. Lumpectomy is a surgical procedure in which the tumor mass and limited surrounding tissues are removed, preserving much of the rest of the breast. Mastectomy is a surgical procedure in which the entire cancerous breast is removed. Over and over, dispassionately, mechanically, I review the words Myron used. They are familiar, part of my medical vocabulary, useful in speaking about patients. Their meaning applies to other people, but not to me.

A nurse practitioner steps into the clinic room to do a preoperative physical examination. No matter what I decide about my surgical treatment, mastectomy or lumpectomy plus radiation, I'm going to have an operation.

When she palpates my ankle pulses, I say, "Ignore the hairy legs."

Her giggle echoes off the examining room walls.

"See, my schedule is to shave my legs in the shower on Sunday mornings." For some reason I feel the need to explain all this to her. "But I was in California last Sunday, so it didn't happen."

She nods. We both know hairy legs don't matter at all, certainly not here, certainly not now.

"I realize this is ridiculous," she says, "but I have to examine your breasts."

"These must be the most examined breasts in the universe," I say. In addition to a mammogram, in the past week I have had five breast exams by five different doctors.

As that nurse leaves, a different nurse enters the examining room. She instructs me about managing the Jackson-Pratt (JP) drain I will have after my axillary dissection. I try to follow what she's saying, but I absolutely don't know why she's teaching this to me at this time.

She dangles the tubing between us and explains its parts.

As I understand it, we don't know yet if I will need to actually *have* an axillary dissection, the operation that would require this tube.

She shows me how to evacuate the bulb.

Am I missing something? Why is she doing this now? I haven't chosen between lumpectomy and mastectomy yet. Between axillary dissection and sentinel node dissection. I just learned about an hour ago that I have cancer, for God's sake.

She tells me something about measuring the drainage in the bulb and calling the Cancer Center if it's over a certain amount.

I can't take in what she's saying. I know I'm mixed up today, but I really don't get it. I am solidly confident, however, that *if* I end up with an axillary dissection, I won't remember a word of this instruction.

I'm back in the radiology waiting room for the second time today. The first was this morning, seemingly a million years ago, for the mammogram; this afternoon I'm here for a chest x-ray. It's another part of the preoperative routine: pre-op physical, done; EKG (because I'm over age fifty), done; blood tests, done; chest x-ray, in progress.

Clusters of people—different from before, but they all look alike—continue to dot the waiting room. The fish still drift in the aquarium with the ease of a whisper, but now their beautiful colors seem muted.

My sense of self hovers in an orbit where it has never been before. I know I have cancer, yet I don't know I have cancer. The word *cancer* spins through my head like a crazed bird—out of context, beyond my reach, unrecognizable, imponderable. It can't find a place to land. It has nothing to do with me.

The radiology clerk calls my name and I hand her the requisition. I've seen—have written—thousands of these forms requesting x-rays. I glance briefly at the paper as I pass it forward. In that fast glimpse, I don't see what I expect. In the rectangle where the reason for the examination is written, it doesn't say "pre-op" or "routine." It doesn't say "55-year-old with breast mass." It says, in bold letters that scream out their meaning, "*R/O mets.*" I stare, disbelieving, at the requisition as the clerk pulls it from my frozen hand.

"Rule out metastases," it says in code. "Rule out metastases." My name and registration number are stamped in the patient ID rectangle. This isn't a mistake. I didn't get someone else's requisition. It's mine.

My hand grabs the edge of the reception desk. Spots, bright and effervescent, flash in front of my face. On the x-ray view box of my mind I see a chest radiograph—two rows of ribs lined up like ladders, a sternum overlying a stack of backbones, a lump of heart. And there, scattered over the black background of the lungs, are fluffy patches as white as dumplings. The dumplings are metastases, islands of cancer growing deep in my lungs.

But, wait, this is all in my mind. I don't have mets yet, at least not that I know of. I have cancer, and this x-ray is part of the preoperative procedure.

# CHAPTER 4

Telling My People

*Our home's back entryway* is as quiet as a crypt, its air still and heavy with the breath of venison stew. Jim has heated a pot of leftovers for dinner.

As I hang my coat in the closet, Cat, Joe's aged tabby, steps out of her litter box and creeps across the wooden floor, past the washer and dryer, past the pantry cupboard, past the shelves of cookbooks. Heading toward her favorite heat register, she seems terribly innocent. She's stuck in her routine and completely unaware of the devastation about to happen around her. The news will crush Jim. He wants to know, needs to know. But my words will be inconceivably awful for him.

I round the corner into the kitchen. From his roost in the La-Z-Boy, Jim stares wide-eyed at me, a giant question mark carved into his face. I move to his side and take his hand. "It's positive."

He closes his eyes, pulls me into his lap, wraps his arms around me. "I knew it would be." His voice is a whisper. "I could tell from the feel of the mass."

After almost thirty years of marriage, I can read his thoughts. I know what grips his senses right now, what paralyzes his reason. It's a childhood memory, a haunting echo he can never escape. He's standing beside his father at the train station in Valley City, North Dakota, waiting for his mother to come home. She has been away, during what would seem like an eternity to a six-year-old, for treatment of her breast cancer. The train chugs to a stop, and his mother steps down to the platform. To her little boy, she looks different than before, thinner, older, gray. When she hugs him, she smells funny, like a burned squirrel. For the rest of his childhood Jim carries that horrible odor, expecting, as everyone in his town does, his mother to die. She doesn't die—five decades later she still hasn't died—and the smell is long gone, except in Jim's subconscious mind. Now he has to go through it all over again with the other woman he loves so deeply.

We sit without speaking, each caught in our own thoughts, both comforted by our togetherness.

"It's ductal carcinoma," I finally say, repeating Myron's words. "We need to decide on lumpectomy or mastectomy."

"The recurrence rates are identical." Jim now uses his surgeon voice. "So the decision hinges on whether or not to retain the breast. After mastectomy, a reconstructed breast is never a beautiful breast, never identical to its mate."

He smooths my hair and tucks a lock behind my ear. He's a chimera—half doctor, half husband. "Radiated breasts aren't entirely normal either."

I'm not a breast-focused woman. My chest appendages aren't who I am. Nursing my sons was rewarding, was fulfilling, but breast-feeding has no relevance to my life decisions now. I have watched my ninety-one-year-old mother-in-law live a full, uncompromised life following a radical mastectomy without reconstruction. Having only one breast wouldn't be unbearable. A mastectomy wouldn't be so bad. I could have Myron lop off the whole cancerous thing and be done with it. And yet, and yet . . .

We keep talking: about scars, about implants, about fat and muscle flaps. We drink a bottle of wine. I'm not ready to make the decision about the surgery yet. It will come, but not quite now.

"Here's what we'll do," Jim says. He and I agree—he will place the telephone call to our son Daniel in Oregon, and after Dan hears the bad news, I will take the phone and reassure him with my upbeat attitude.

"Hi, Dan." Jim's voice is a cheerful masquerade. "How's work?" He nods at Daniel's answer and then describes the bamboo fly rod he wants to build.

"How's Bean?" Jim asks. Apparently Dan says something funny about his wife. Jim laughs. He details plans for a fishing trip to Bermuda this summer. They discuss Cuban cigars. Suddenly the small talk stops.

Jim stares at me, his eyes desperate. "Ah, Dan . . ." His voice has lost its mask; it's heavy, dark. I watch his eyes tear. His moist lashes beat together, trying to erase the dampness.

"Dan." Our son's name comes out thick, as if it bubbled through a pile of oatmeal. "Your mom has something to tell you." Jim hands me the phone and a sob escapes from deep inside him.

"Honey," I say to Dan. This is easier for me than for Jim. I ache to speak with our child-now-a-man, to explain the thing that smothers me, to draw him into a tight ring of caring people around me. "I need to tell you what has just entered my life."

"What, Mom?" Dan is puzzled and worried. I can tell from the tiny quiver in his voice, from the way he clips his words.

"Breast cancer."

"You're kidding."

"No, honey, I'm not kidding. It's for real."

"Hi, Nancy. It's me." Nancy is my sister, fourteen months my junior. She, like Daniel, lives three time zones away in Portland, Oregon.

I tell her about my cancer. She's stunned but calm.

I'm the classic older sibling, the guardian, the boss. I remember Nancy as a little girl sobbing to our mother in the kitchen of our tiny rental house in Fargo, "No matter how old I am, Janet will always be older."

She was right. I'm always older: first to graduate from high school and college, first to marry, first to have a child. And now, first to have cancer.

"I need you to do a huge favor for me," I say.

"What?"

I know she will do whatever I ask. "Please call Mom and Dad and tell them."

In the background her dogs are barking and her daughter is yelling to shut them up. "You don't want to?" Nancy asks.

"No. I have too much to take care of right now. I can't take care of them as well."

"OK. I'll call them tonight. They'll be pretty upset, you know."

"I know."

Nancy understands. She has a different relationship with our parents than I do and plays a different role in the theater of our family. I'm the strong, smart, responsible daughter; she's the fun-loving, easy-going one.

Telling Joe, who continues to express his independence by keeping his distance from us, is a logistical nightmare. Since he has no telephone—uses the pay phone down the hallway in the barracks to call out—I have no way to contact him except by the U.S. Postal Service. His e-mail account is one of those off-and-on-again deals, and he hasn't answered my last several messages. Besides, I want to tell him in a more personal way than through cyberspace, so I compose a letter. I explain that my doctor found a mass in my breast, that the biopsy showed it was cancer. The note is cheerful, matter-of-fact. I tell him that I will have an operation and remind him that his Grandma Gilsdorf had breast cancer fifty years ago and is still a vibrant, crazy lady. She's the woman with the wandering boob, for her foam prosthesis seems to roam all over her chest. My final instructions in the letter are to call home immediately.

It's now two days since he should have received that letter; I sent it by overnight mail. We've heard nothing from him, but we know he doesn't check his mailbox very often. I'm irritated. I want to talk to him, to reassure him, to gather him, also, into the tight ring of supporters around me. I wish he wouldn't keep himself so isolated. Why haven't I insisted he give us the number to that pay phone?

Google is a godsend. Through an electronic search I identify the Defense Language Institute Web site, find the link to the United States Navy command, and, finally, locate a phone number for the Officer of the Day. He, I assume, is the guy on call, the fellow who handles all the unexpected stuff.

A pleasant, polite young man answers the phone. His voice is as clean and sharply creased as I imagine his dress-white navy uniform to be.

"This is Janet Gilsdorf from Ann Arbor, Michigan. I'm trying to reach my son Joe Gilsdorf about a family situation. He's in the French program, in the navy."

"Ma'am," the Officer of the Day says, "would you please spell his name?"

"G-I-L-S-D-O-R-F. Joseph. Could someone stick a note on his door telling him to call home?"

"Yes, ma'am. I'll send someone over there right away."

Less than an hour later, Jim and I are discussing how to tell his mother about my cancer when the phone rings.

"Hi, Mom." It's Joe.

"Honey." A gasp of relief gushes from me. "I have something important to tell you."

"Yeah, Mom, I know. I just read your letter."

My cancer will be hard for Joe. He's young, a guy without sisters, and still mystified by womanly things, especially female body parts. I'm sure a discussion of his mother's breasts makes him uncomfortable. Worst of all, he is far away and alone. Dan has a wonderful wife who will help him through this. Joe has no one but Jim and me.

Too soon it's time to say good-bye. I long to give Joe a hug; I wish he could see my face to know that I'm OK. "Honey, this is a big jolt for you."

"Remember, Mom, I listened to you and dad talk about medical junk the whole time I was growing up." He's forever the tough guy.

"Yes, but this 'medical junk' involves your mom."

If I could see him, I'd watch him shrug.

"Joe, you might want to talk about this with someone. A chaplain might work. They know how to help guys through rough places." I'm not speaking from strong religious convictions, because I have none. Rather, I'm remembering Joe's story about the camel ride while his ship was docked in Jebel Ali, in the United Arab Emirates. The outing was organized by the USS *Samuel Gompers'* recreation director, a chaplain. "I assume the institute has a chaplain or two around."

"Mom, I'm fine."

To me, the Henry F. Vaughan School of Public Health building is a grande dame of a structure, with tall ceilings, oak cabinets, brass fixtures, and marble stalls in the bathrooms. She holds many secrets, including the celebration my research group staged after we cloned the *Haemophilus influenzae* pilin gene. One of the overhead tiles still bears the divot from the champagne bottle's cork. To set the record straight, serving alcohol in this building is forbidden in accordance with university bylaws.

My research laboratory is here, clustered alongside my colleagues' labs in the Center for Molecular and Clinical Epidemiology of Infectious Diseases. Betsy the epidemiologist, Carl the microbiologist, and I the physician scientist are ideal scientific collaborators, with complementary individual strengths. We share everything: research funds, graduate students, laboratory equipment, reagents, and ideas for novel projects. Now we need to share my bad news.

I've asked them to meet me in Carl's office. Leafless vines drape the outside of the sole, dusty window, and, beyond, a patch of grass is barely visible beneath a brick wall. A lacy spiderweb clings to the corner of the window frame; its delicate silver strands shimmer in the sunlight. We sit like three points of a triangle surrounded by filing cabinets and bookshelves. My body language must scream "trouble," because both Carl and Betsy are guarded.

"I need to tell you my new situation." My words are stiff, formal for such close, dear colleagues. "I've just learned that I have breast cancer." Betsy's face twists as if she is about to cry. Carl can't speak, silenced by emotion. They both give me hugs.

I have never felt their bodies before now. In our work, we touch each other academically, intellectually, creatively, but never physically. Through the fabric of their shirts their back muscles are taut against my palms. The warmth from their skin on my skin hints of an indiscretion, a misdeed, a tiny sin. Yet, their heat, their aliveness, is comforting.

My cancer has moved us into foreign territory. Betsy and Carl will do as they always have done, but more so now; they will assist my students and technicians, cover the gap, be there.

✿

My brother, the color-blind paint chemist from Houston, Texas, calls. He's heard the news from our sister Nancy.

"Now, take it easy," he says. "You have a pretty bad track record for relaxing."

"Me?" I feign surprise. "You must have mistaken me for someone else."

"Just remember," he jests, "our sister Nancy—the one who used to cheat in Monopoly—would be using this for all it's worth. Maybe you should try a little of that."

✿

They are all men, the other four faculty members of the Pediatric Infectious Diseases division, and they are bewildered. Never before have I summoned them together to my office. Not knowing what to expect, they crowd into the small room, anxiously shoving borrowed chairs into the limited space.

When I tell them I have breast cancer, they gasp in unison. I may be a woman, but I'm their leader and they see me as strong and invincible. They are all pediatricians and know about malignancies, but hearing about mine unnerves them. They look like a row of worried boys facing a mighty, but injured, mother.

I've prepared for this meeting, have all my cards aligned. I tell them that I've discussed my illness with the chairman of the department and that he will not appoint an acting director. Rather, I will continue my administrative duties to the division. I assure them that if I can't fulfill these responsibilities, the decision about leadership will be reconsidered. They nod.

I tell them I won't be able to be the attending physician on the Pediatric Infectious Diseases consultation service in April as scheduled and that Graham, John, and Alex will each cover ten April days. They can decide among themselves who does which segment. They nod.

I tell them I can't be certain what my treatment will entail, so the next several months will be in limbo. I ask them to be flexible, knowing that they can and will. They nod.

Finally, I tell them that my cancer is not a secret, that I will depend on the rumor mill to get the word to the postdoctoral fellows, that I have a meeting with the administrative staff later this morning.

Alex raises his hand, as if he's in fourth grade. "We'll take care of revising the clinical service schedule," he says. "You take care of yourself. You would have done the same for any of us."

There isn't a better group of colleagues anywhere.

Bean, my daughter-in-law, sends me a care package. It contains a tofu cookbook, mango tea, apricot skin lotion, plum-flavored sugarless candy, and a colorful box of aromatherapy bath salts. I've never had a daughter, have lived my adult life in a household of males. Bean comes from a family of women who are skilled at mending many kinds of hurts.

Even though I'm a shower rather than a bath person and less into naturopathic healing than Bean is, I treasure these gifts. They are her thoughtful way of soothing me, of easing the discomfort, psychic and otherwise.

The package also contains a note in Daniel's breezy handwriting that says, "Mom, I know you don't take many baths, but you should."

When I call to thank them, Daniel says, "I don't want to dismiss your illness, but compared to the medical horror stories we've heard from you and Dad over the years, this seems relatively easy."

Two days later he calls back. "Mom, it's bothering me a lot more than I expected."

Tom's office is two doors down the hallway from mine. He will vacate it soon, however, as he is about to retire. We already have plans for this office. The divisional secretary will move here so she can have a window, and her long, narrow, dingy office will turn into a postdoctoral fellows' room. At the university, your desk seat hasn't cooled before it's reassigned.

Tom's office is appointed with relics of the two decades he has spent on the faculty, the personal touches that reflect his humanness in an otherwise institutional room. There in the corner is the Windsor chair with the seal of the medical school on the headrest—his reward for serving as associate dean of student affairs. On the file cabinet stands a Thai dancing doll, her six arms waving a seductive hello. His EIS (Epidemic Intelligence Service) certificate in its austere government frame hangs between the window and a bookshelf. Predominantly, on his desk, a faded picture of his father, a noted virologist who inspired his three sons to become virologists, is flanked by decades-old photos of Tom's smiling wife and three impish children.

I'm here to see if Tom would consider delaying his retirement for a few months. I need to find a way to cover the Pediatric Infectious Diseases consultation service responsibilities if I require chemotherapy. The rest of the Pediatric Infectious Diseases faculty can each do a bit more, but we will need additional help.

From time to time for almost twenty years Tom and I have discussed patients in either my office or his—summarizing cases as we pass the baton of the clinical service from one to the other, asking an opinion about a diagnostic or therapeutic dilemma, sharing the interesting details of an unusual infection. There was the beautiful cheerleader who died of mono; the Amish baby boy whose eight older siblings had died of the same disorder that was killing him; the girl with rabies; the lad with bad encephalitis who suddenly woke up and demanded an ice cream cone. Many, many times I have stared into this thin handsome face framed by professorial gray hair, into these glimmering blue eyes. As always, his signature bow tie rests far beneath his chin.

I explain my situation; detail the upcoming surgical procedures and radiation therapy, the possible chemotherapy; describe the characteristics of the tumor. I'm using our medical language, the words we have exchanged at least weekly. They fall from my lips as easily as spring rain: neoplasm, FNA, metatastasis, pre-op, post-op.

Suddenly, the reality of my words hits me like an avalanche. I'm talking about me. Not a patient. Me. These medical details are mine, written in my record, sticking to my tissues, incorporated into my being. They're not attached to another person with a different name, age, gender, registration number, or diagnosis.

A weird, out-of-body sensation, smooth and stealthy as a gray silk drape, sweeps through my mind. A part of me hovers near the ceiling of Tom's office, watching him nod and scratch his arm while he listens to a lady doctor discussing a patient. From afar, I see the two of us talking. The words coming from the lady doctor are *my* words, are about me.

Slowly, like a spirit coming home, I return to reality, to my body seated on the chair, to the person speaking with Tom. He agrees to delay his retirement if necessary.

My current journal is a small legal pad inside a notebook cover made of Atlantic salmon skin that I bought on the Gaspé Peninsula of Quebec. On a lemon-colored page I write,

> *If I have to go into the hospital for a while, I'll . . .*
> * *Wear a white, lacy nightgown.*
> * *Take my French-milled soap and make the nurses bathe me with it.*
> * *Order fresh flowers every day.*
> * *Take my homemade lap robe.*

Joe calls again.

"What's the matter, honey?" I ask. "You don't sound so good."

"Hey, man. I'm worried about you." His voice is strained. "It's rough when Mom's down."

"Janet?" my sister Nancy asks over the phone. "I can't remember the name of what you have. Duck melamoma or something like that."

"Ductal carcinoma."

"Duck serumoma?"

"Ductal carcinoma."

"Duck carcinoloma?"

"Nancy, why don't you just call it 'breast cancer'?"

"Oh, no," she gasps. "That sounds too bad."

"Mom."

It's Joe, again, on the phone from Monterey.

"Hi, honey."

"Mom, I want to come home for your operation."

"You'll have to miss class. Is it worth that?"

"It is to me. I've talked to my teachers and have gotten the assignments for those days. I can work on them in Ann Arbor."

Since I can't actually touch him, I caress what will eventually rest in his hands—the envelope addressed to him and wedged between the phone and the fruit bowl. Inside are cartoons and fun pictures and interesting stories cut from newspapers and magazines. Throughout his time in the navy, I've sent similar envelopes to him.

He continues, "I need you to do something for me. I'm requesting an emergency family leave. You need to call the Red Cross and give them the information about your operation so my chief will let me off."

"Sure, whatever it takes. Do I just call the Ann Arbor Red Cross? The place where you donate blood?"

"I guess so. Wherever the closest Red Cross office is."

There's only one number in the phone book for the American Red Cross. Indeed, it's the place where blood donations are taken.

I introduce myself to the man who answers the phone and explain what I need.

"OK, ma'am," he says. "I have a few questions for you."

He asks for my phone number. He asks for my doctor's name and phone number.

"That's it, ma'am. I'll get in touch with your son's command right away."

"Nothing else?"

"No, ma'am. That's all I need."

Two hours later, Joe calls again.

"Mom, I just got authorization for the leave. I'll be there Thursday night."

I'm amazed. I wouldn't have guessed that anything in the military, in the entire federal government, could work so smoothly.

※

Last week I walked the halls of this hospital as a staff physician. Now, as I return to my office from a meeting, I'm a patient. The hallways look different. I notice things I've never seen before. Those benches below the windows across from the transfusion office, the purple faux leather seats with splayed maple legs. How long have they been there? And the courtyard is different, more serene. The tree skeletons sway gently in the wind; the swollen tips of their twigs are asleep, waiting for a springtime signal to erupt into baby leaves. I ride the elevator up one level and walk under the glass canopy to the children's hospital; the windows are streaky from past rain showers. Beyond the unisex bathroom I turn into the Pediatric Infectious Diseases offices. The scenery is familiar, but I see it now through new eyes, process it through a new mind.

Even the people in the corridor look different. The doctors, my colleagues and friends, hustle past. What's their hurry? They nod, smile, mutter "hello." They have no idea I'm not the same person they saw last week. Patients, wrapped in their winter coats, amble through the halls gazing at the room numbers, then at the maps and instruction sheets clutched in their hands. I'm a patient, too, now. Do I appear as lost as they are?

Outside, the February sun warms the pavement and melts the last remnants of snow. I'm driving away from the hospital and suddenly have no idea how I got to the car. I have no recollection of the walk from my office to the parking garage, no memory of the search for my blue Dodge Spirit.

Next thing I know, I'm turning into the parking lot at Busch's grocery store. Why am I here? I haven't been thinking about groceries. But, then, I'm not sure what I've been thinking.

Several months ago I crossed paths with a woman I hadn't seen for a while.

"Nice haircut," I said, referring to her pert, short new look that had replaced her shoulder-length old look.

"Oh," she said, "that's my breast cancer-do."

I was shocked, had no idea she had been treated for cancer. She made a sour face and scurried off.

Now I want to speak with her. She's a physician, so we share the Janus-like perspective of being a doctor and a patient. Amazingly, very few women I know well have been through breast cancer. No family members. No close friends. I call her, and we agree to meet this afternoon.

Her hair is very short, a mass of twisted gray wires. She says that chemo just about killed her, although she gained ten pounds from the steroids and from lying around doing nothing.

"Look at this." She holds out her arms. "See the puffiness?" She flaps her left hand and tugs at her wedding ring. "Lymphedema from the axillary dissection. It's ugly and increases my risk of lymphoma. If this happens to you, I recommend Rhonda in Occupational Therapy. She's great." Step by step, my friend walks the fingers of her left hand up an imaginary wall, demonstrating one of her shoulder exercises.

"After my axillary dissection, my husband had to come home every noon to strip my JP drain." She itemizes her complaints. "I hate the Cancer Center. Hate the icy nurses, hate the walls, hate the floor, hate the ceiling, hate the infusion chairs, hate the windows, hate every single thing about the place.

"I had to give myself G-CSF (granulocyte colony stimulating factor) injections for neutropenia. I was so scared of getting an infection that I constantly walked around the house with a box of alcohol wipes, compulsively scrubbing the refrigerator handle and the faucet knobs and the phone receiver.

"The first four weeks of radiation weren't too bad—nothing like the chemo—but I was totally exhausted the last two weeks.

"I took seven months off work, figured for once I needed to take care of myself. 'Screw the system,' I said. 'They'll find a way to get along without me.'

"Hot flashes from menopause are nothing compared to the tamoxifen hot flashes. Four, five, six times a night I soak the sheets. And, of course, tamoxifen increases my risk of uterine cancer.

"The Cancer Center has a wig bank, but forget it. I never had any company at home so I just stayed bald. When I went to the store or to the hospital for infusions or blood draws or radiation, I just tied a scarf around my bare head."

Her final comment is, "Welcome to the sorority."

Sorority. That word haunts me. A club of women. I was never good at sororities.

When I was growing up in North Dakota, girls didn't become doctors. Rather, they became nurses or teachers or social workers, but that was just temporary because, most important of all, they became wives and mothers.

But I was different. I wanted to do something important with my life, to make an impact on the world. *Arrowsmith* was my favorite book, and Dr. Tom Dooley was my hero. He was a physician who established medical facilities in Southeast Asia and died at age thirty-four of malignant melanoma. Years later, I learned, to my deep disappointment, that he was, in reality, quite the charlatan. In college, I joined

Kappa Alpha Theta because becoming a sorority pledge was the thing to do. Increasingly, I grew apart from my sorority sisters. They worked hard to land husbands while I worked hard for good grades to get into medical school. Some of my closest friends at North Dakota State University were nonsorority women who were biology and pharmacy majors and, thus, somewhat oddballs themselves.

At the University of North Dakota Medical School, I was the only woman in my class of 42 students to finish the first two years. I then transferred to the University of Nebraska, where my class of 130 students included three women. For years I had only a few women friends, and they were the rare other women physicians. We didn't play bridge or golf or go shopping or enjoy leisurely lunches. We worked all the time and had no regrets.

Nurses, all women then, were sometimes just plain hostile, and several of my classmates and professors, all men, were very cruel. Fortunately, the gender landscape in medicine is different now; 40–50 percent of medical students are women, and men increasingly choose to become nurses. But, among doctors my age, the old imbalance still applies.

Now, it appears, I'm in a different kind of sorority, one whose pledges get fine needle aspirates, lumpectomies, and axillary dissections. Full members get chemotherapy, radiation, or five years of tamoxifen. Alumnae get lymphedema, metastases or secondary malignancies. Breast cancer sorority sisters wile away the hours in the hospital waiting rooms reading ragged, outdated *Good Housekeeping* magazines—Christmas issue in April, Halloween issue in January. Their uniform includes scarves, wigs or hats, and hospital gowns.

The injustice of it all is maddening. I lived much of my adult life as a woman in a man's world, a lady doctor in the male-dominated universe of medicine. How many times have I been the only woman in a meeting except for the secretary who takes notes and makes coffee? Suddenly I'm a woman with a woman's disease. It's cruel to have cancer but, for me, far crueler to have a woman's cancer. In our society, womanly things are undervalued, overlooked, ridiculed. I don't want to carry the stain of a woman's illness, too. If I have to have cancer, why can't I have an astrocytoma or osteosarcoma or lymphoma—any kind of gender-neutral malignancy? I don't like this sorority and don't want to be part of the sisterhood. Somehow it feels like a demotion.

My physician friend's bitterness about her cancer reeks like black bile, and even now, over a year after her diagnosis, she boils with anger.

"I don't think I can do this," I whisper to myself. Never before in my life have I viewed anything as impossible.

# Chapter 5

*"Lies, damn lies, and statistics"*

— BENJAMIN DISRAELI —

*"You can't have breast cancer, Janet,"* my sister Patty says.

"Well, I do." We are speaking by telephone, but in my mind's eye I see the grimace on her disbelieving face.

"No one in our family has ever had breast cancer."

She's right. No one in our family has had breast cancer, but that may be misleading because we have a shortage of women. I have only two sisters and three female cousins, all younger. We have no blood aunts, as our mother was an only child and our father had three brothers. According to Mother, the family historian, neither of our grandmothers and none of their sisters had breast cancer. One great-grandmother may have died of "throat cancer." She couldn't swallow and starved to death. Another died of "old age." She was blind and reportedly ate a fair number of ants along with her stale cakes and sandwiches, but having too many birthdays was what killed her. I come from sturdy, northern European immigrants who lived long lives in spite of—or because of—Minnesota winters.

So, what about families and breast cancer? The likelihood of developing certain types of cancer is inherited, and the risk is a numbers game, not unlike blackjack. Instead of the luck of the draw, though, cancers depend on the luck of the genes. About 5 percent of breast cancers occur because of mutations in genes called BRCA1 (named for BReast CAncer) or BRCA2. Such genes normally instruct cells to make tumor suppressor proteins, the molecular monitors that tell breast cells when to stop growing. Mutations, or genetic mistakes, in tumor suppressor genes turn them from the "on" mode—making suppressor proteins—to the "off" mode—not making suppressor proteins. In the absence of suppressor proteins, cells with mutations in BRCA1 or BRCA2 genes don't die but keep growing. And growing. And growing. The end result is cancer.

I don't know if I carry this gene. It's unlikely because of my pristine family history and the fact that my ancestors are Scandinavians, Scots, and Germans rather than Ashkenazi Jews, who are much more likely than other ethnic groups to carry mutations in BRCA1 or BRCA2. Besides, these genetic mistakes only account for one in twenty cases of breast cancer.

So, why did I get mine? In addition to mutated genes, there are other factors that increase, although to a lesser degree, the risk of developing breast cancer. It's tempting to keep score.

- Over forty years old? Yes
- Affluent? I don't think we *live* affluently, if that's the issue. We have a nice home but not a castle. Most of our furniture is hand-me-downs from my mother-in-law or crafted by my husband. I knit our sweaters and buy many of our clothes on sale. Obviously, with two physicians in the family, our household income is well above average. I guess we score high on the affluence scale.
- Born in a cold climate? Yes. Minneapolis clearly has a cold climate.
- Born in the Western Hemisphere? Yes, again.
- Caucasian? Yes
- Fibrocystic changes in the breast? Yes.
- Sedentary lifestyle? Unfortunately, yes. My vocation as an academic physician and scientist requires much more cerebral work than physical work, and my avocation is writing, very much a sit-down activity.
- Tall? Maybe. I'm five feet, five inches in height.
- High body fat? Maybe. I think of myself as "pleasantly plump." This is a risk factor because estrogen is stored in fat. Obese women have more estrogen in their bodies than skinny women, and estrogen feeds some breast cancers.
- Use of alcohol? Yes, a glass of wine with dinner. That's my

heart medicine—moderate intake of alcohol may reduce my
risk of coronary artery disease. What's a person to do about
conflicting risk factors? Would I rather have a heart attack
than breast cancer? I don't like these choices. I'd rather have
neither.

- Menarche before age twelve? Late menopause? Nulliparous
(meaning never having been pregnant)? Delivered first child
after age thirty? No, no, no, and no. Daniel was born when I
was almost twenty-eight. These risk factors all have to do
with prolonged exposure to estrogen.

- Exogenous estrogens? Yes, I took hormone replacement
therapy, but for only three years. The risk for breast cancer
seems to increase after five years of use. In a study of nurses,
the relative risk of breast cancer among women on HRTs
was 1.36, meaning that users were 1.36 times more likely
than nonusers to get breast cancer. To say this another way,
if my inherent risk of getting breast cancer was 2.0 percent,
taking HRTs would increase that risk to 2.72 percent. In
truth, of course, it's more complicated than that—real risk
figures are elusive, sometimes twisting, sometimes darting
targets. To be more accurate, you need to factor in the risk
differences at various ages and the length of time HRTs are
used. In any event, while taking HRTs increases the risk of
breast cancer, the magnitude of the increased risk is small.

It's impossible to know how these findings apply to me or to any
single individual. At best, they describe an average risk over hundreds
of women, and the biology of my body isn't identical to those other
hundreds. Considering that the risk of breast cancer from taking HRTs
is low, that it is only one of many intertwined risk factors, that my decision to take them was based on the best information at the time, and
that without HRTs I wouldn't have been able to do my work, I have *no
regrets* about taking hormone replacement therapy. Thank goodness.
Being stalked by the "if onlys" is a terrible way to live.

Breast cancer is common. Women in the United States have a
12–13 percent chance of getting it during their lifetime, which trans-

lates into a probability of one in eight, if they live to be 110 years old! The longer you live, the higher the likelihood of being diagnosed with breast cancer; older women are more likely to develop this disease than younger women. For a woman like me, with few risk factors and no family history, the chance that I would get breast cancer between ages fifty and sixty years is one in sixty-three. If I had two sisters with breast cancer, the chance would skyrocket to one in eight.

Consider the statistics among members of my writing group—one (me) in five; among members of my book group—one (me) in six; among the women of my generation in my family—one (me) in six. What about the others in these groups? I've told them that since I have it, they don't need to get it. I'm the token victim in each cohort. I sincerely hope that's true.

Why did I get breast cancer? Did I do something wrong? Am I bad? Is there some reason I was selected to have this disease? Am I being punished for a moment of cosmic sin? For a year of indiscretion? For a lifetime of poor judgment?

At the end of the day, the reason for my cancer remains a secret buried deep in my chromosomes, possibly enabled at some small step along the way by a nudge from my environment. For whatever reason, one cell in one of my left milk ducts made a genetic mistake. It was a DNA typo, a slipup, a wrong turn into a one-way street, a shattered goblet, a broken promise, a cinder that jumped from the fire to the carpet and set the whole room ablaze.

The oak and apple logs snap as they burn, and the flames from the fireplace lend serenity to the room. I'm tucked into my overstuffed chair, and Jim is tipped back in his La-Z-Boy. Outside, the February wind blows the snowflakes sideways at a forty-five-degree angle. Jim is reviewing the cancer survival and recurrence statistics for me. I need to decide between mastectomy or lumpectomy plus radiation.

"The goal is to control local disease in the breast," he says. He's using his surgeon voice again, speaking as if I'm on the examining table and he's in his white coat. That's OK, because I need the information. Yesterday I searched the MedLine electronic database of medical literature and found a series of articles in the *Surgical Clinics of North America* that review the management of breast cancer. I printed a copy. To be able to make my decision about an operation, I need a context, a sense of the biology of breast cancer, a refresher course on the principles of surgical therapy for this disease.

"You're a good candidate for breast conservation therapy"— that's lumpectomy plus radiation—"because of the relatively small size of your tumor," Jim says, "and its location and the relatively large size of your breast."

36C. The ample shelf that catches cookie crumbs and coffee drizzles now allows me a few options.

"How about lumpectomy alone and skip the radiation?" I ask.

"That's a no-go. Lumpectomy alone results in a 25 to 40 percent chance of recurrence in that breast."

Of course. The cancer may not be limited to the little almond that we feel, to the lump that would be removed during the lumpectomy. Rather, residual cancer cells may lurk in the lymphatic channels that track like a spider web through the rest of my breast tissue.

He tells me the most important statistic in my decision making. "The survival rates after a decade are essentially the same," he says. "Sixty percent after mastectomy and 62 percent after lumpectomy."

"So . . . ," I say, quickly doing the math in my head, ". . . a death rate of 40 percent versus 38 percent in ten years." The fire has quit snapping. It needs another log. "That's pretty crappy."

"Some of those women, especially the older women, die for other reasons, you know."

Of course, again. Breast cancer isn't the only cause of death in those who get it. "I'm going to live until I'm at least eighty-five," I say.

"That's right," my husband agrees.

The difference between 60 percent and 62 percent—survival rates after mastectomy or lumpectomy plus radiation, respectively—is meaningless. It's within biologic variation. If you toss a quarter ten times, you might get four heads and six tails. If you do it again with the same quarter, you might get six heads and four tails. There is no difference between 40 percent heads and 60 percent heads when you toss

*"Lies, damn lies, and statistics"*

the coin so few times. The difference in these numbers can be explained by chance. Similarly, the small difference between 60 percent and 62 percent in breast cancer survival rates is most likely caused by chance or, more realistically, by unknown biologic differences among the women who participated in the studies.

In considering my options, the survival difference is chump change. Still, relying on the subjective calculator deep within my gut rather than the objective one in my head, the bigger survival number in the lumpectomy group stays with me.

Jim throws another hunk of apple wood on the fire and rearranges the glowing embers with the poker.

My mind can't lock on images that depict my options. I haven't seen many reconstructed breasts or many postlumpectomy or postradiation breasts. I have, however, seen post–radical mastectomy chests. My mother-in-law has one, as did several patients when I was in medical school and one of the cadavers in my gross anatomy class. As these mental pictures march through my head, the retention of part of my own breast seems more appealing than having no breast, with or without the patch-up of a reconstruction.

"Should we go for lumpectomy and radiation, then?" I ask Jim. It's a rhetorical question, meant to fill the otherwise quiet air with sound.

"It's up to you, honey. It's your body."

Even though he's right and I wouldn't want him to say anything else, I need a partner in this. I don't want to drive this out-of-control bus all alone. I want someone to tell me my choice is a good one.

"Yeah," I nod. "But since you're the expert, I want you to agree with me."

"I agree."

The next decision concerns the method to detect whether my cancer has already spread beyond the firm almond in my breast. The choices are sentinel node mapping, a minor procedure in which one to several lymph nodes are surgically removed from the armpit, or axillary node dissection, a major operation in which many lymph nodes are removed. In either case, the removed nodes are examined for malignant cells because spread of the cancer to the lymph nodes is predictive of—but not necessarily the first step in—spread to other regions of the body. In addition, the number of positive nodes, those containing cancer, is used to determine the potential value of chemotherapy. To my irrational thinking, in spite of studies showing similar outcomes for both procedures, cutting out cancerous nodes simply seems to be a good idea. Like pulling dandelions. Like scraping mold off the cheese.

In determining the extent of breast cancer, sentinel node mapping is a relatively new alternative to axillary dissection. During the mapping procedure two markers, a blue dye and a radioactive tracer, are injected directly into the tumor. The markers travel away from the cancer through lymphatic channels and puddle in the first lymph node they encounter—the "sentinel node," which will be surgically removed. First a nuclear medicine scan indicates that the tracer has reached a node, and then in the operating room a Geiger counter is used to detail its general location. Finally, through a small incision lateral to the breast, the surgeon identifies and removes the blue-tinted node, which is sent to the laboratory, where pathologists examine it for cancer cells.

My surgeon had explained that the doctors at the Cancer Center have been doing sentinel node mapping for several years. Studies have shown it to be 95 percent accurate in predicting spread of the cancer to nearby lymph nodes.

Ninety-five percent. That's not 100 percent. So, if the sentinel node is negative, there's still a 5 percent chance that I have at least one positive axillary node, which translates to a one in twenty chance that my treatment plan might be based on inaccurate data. My surgeon didn't mention the 5 percent part. He didn't have to. I can do the subtraction myself.

"Jim, what do you think about sentinel node biopsy?"

"It's still experimental."

"That's what Myron said. He says the university has had good experience with it."

"Again, honey, the decision is yours."

That's a problem. Right now I don't want to make these kinds of decisions. I want someone to tell me what will be done and that it's absolutely the right thing to do. I'll take the word of someone who is experienced and knowledgeable and who has no other stake in the process than the best medical care for me. Either my surgeon or Jim qualifies as that someone. And neither of them will dictate the route I should go.

I don't like either option. What I really want to do is go to the northern California coast and forget about the whole cancer deal. But I have work to do, a decision to make.

The advantage of sentinel node biopsy is that it could save me from undergoing a complete axillary dissection, with its potential aftereffects. The disadvantage is the small chance—5 percent—that it gives wrong information. In some moments this decision seems like the most critical crossroad I have ever faced, more important than my decision to go to medical school or to marry or to have children. At these times, life or death seems to drift over my head like the shadow of a buzzard. In other moments the decision seems as inconsequential as choosing fried or barbequed chicken for lunch—either would be fine and I'll adjust to the outcome.

How does one make a rational choice? Flip a quarter? Pull straws? Tear the petals off a daisy?

To hell with rationality. I'll take the sentinel node biopsy.

# TWO / The Three Hells

*Surgery*

*Chemotherapy*

*Radiation*

# CHAPTER 6

*Biology for Artists and Linguists*

*After dinner my sons,* Dan visiting from Oregon and Joe from California, help clean the kitchen. My lumpectomy is tomorrow morning, and I want them to understand what's happening to me.

"So, ask me about my cancer or the surgery or whatever," I say as I stack the glasses in the dishwasher.

"No questions," says Daniel.

"I know all about it," says Joe with a sneer and a swagger. "Remember, I grew up in this house hearing the gory stories and seeing the gruesome pictures in your magazines. I know everything I need to know about operations."

What did we do to our sons while they were growing up? They seem to have a hands-off approach to everything medical. After listening to the dinner table descriptions of their parents' professional lives, maybe they can't understand that their mother's sickness is different from her patients' sicknesses, at least in how our family reacts to it.

As the boys would tell you, I can't leave anything alone. I keep picking at this scab. "Well, you may want to know about the surgery—what they'll do and why . . ."

"I've heard it a million times and don't need to hear it again," Joe interrupts.

My sons' responses irritate me. I'm trying to be open with them, and they prefer to remain shut. They think that by keeping out the facts they can keep out the bad feelings. Besides, they are adults now and will need to take responsibility for their own health decisions, so they better get used to these unpleasant conversations. Maybe if I perch on a stool, stay grounded instead of fluttering about the kitchen, they will realize I'm serious about this discussion.

"Well, you should at least know what cancer is," I say. "It's part of being an informed person. It's one course in the curriculum of life."

Daniel hangs his dishtowel on the cabinet door, rests his elbows on the counter, leans his sweet face toward me, and, staring though his wise, sea-blue eyes set deep in their sockets, says, "Well, yes, I guess you could tell me what cancer is."

Joe shuts the refrigerator door and echoes, "Yeah, what *is* cancer, anyway?"

Neither of our sons is inclined toward science. Dan majored in art and earned a Bachelor of Fine Arts degree, with honors, from the University of Colorado. Besides being a sculptor (which *doesn't* pay the bills), he owns a body art shop in Portland and is a very successful tattoo artist (which *does* pay the bills). Joe is a linguist—learning French in the military so he can work in navy intelligence. During a brief college stint, he enrolled in both a German and a Russian course. "Don't be so hard on yourself," I said at the time. "Take one or the other."

His eyes glowered as he replied, "I would much rather take two language classes than one science course!"

"Well," I say, wiping grease off the coffee grinder with a napkin, "cancer refers to cells that are out of control."

In what must sound to them like a graduate seminar in biology, I explain the thing that is growing inside me. ". . . genetic script . . ." ". . . life cycle of a cell . . ." ". . . quality-control police . . ." ". . . molecular monitors that orchestrate the biologic movements in the symphony of life: birth, growth, productive maturity, senescence, death." I'm a professor and a doctor, after all. I clarify medical concepts to people—to my patients, my students, my sons—using words such as these.

"Sometimes the genes that make the monitors get screwed up." I plow ahead with my lecture. "The faulty genes are called oncogenes—'onco' meaning cancer. Oncogenes promote the development of cancer."

"What can screw up the monitor genes and turn them into oncogenes?" I, the Socratic teacher, ask. Before my audience—my two sons—can respond, I answer, "Lots of things."

Joe reaches into the fruit bowl for an orange and begins ripping off the peel.

"Viruses can," I continue. "Certain viruses can stick their own genes into the monitor genes and scramble their message.

"Radiation can. Energy waves such as x-rays or ultraviolet light in huge doses damage DNA.

"Environmental compounds can. Toxins such as asbestos and the trash in tobacco smoke damage cells.

"Lots of time the monitor genes are messed up because of a genetic misstep that happens when the cells are dividing. It's like substituting salt for sugar when making a flan. They are both white and granular and are found in the kitchen cupboard, but the end product just isn't the same."

Dan and Joe glance at each other and smile, undoubtedly remembering a few of the cooking disasters that have occurred in this kitchen.

"The result? When a cell's monitor genes are screwed up, the cell doesn't get the normal signals to slow down, so it keeps growing and dividing. In short, the cell doesn't die. Rather, it keeps on reproducing as if it's immortal—one cell becomes two, which become four, which become eight, on and on. The cluster of abnormal cells enlarges and turns into a tumor, which gets bigger and bigger and invades the normal tissues around it."

Daniel sets the lid on the butter dish to protect it from Cat.

"Apparently my enzymes, metabolic pathways, intercellular signals, or hormones conspired against my well-being and spawned a cell that escaped the molecular monitors, that refused to die according to its molecular script, that kept reproducing and finally became the seed of a tumor nestled in my left breast."

"Ultimately," I say, stepping into scary territory for all of us, "a few cancer cells may break off from the tumor and travel through my blood or lymph channels to other places in my body, and the process may start all over again—one cell becomes two, two become four, et cetera. When this happens, breast cancer shows up in the lymph nodes of the armpit, in lungs, bones, brain, or liver. We hope that hasn't happened to me. We hope my cancer is only in my breast."

Dan fidgets with a can opener; Joe twirls a corkscrew.

"The surgery and radiation will get rid of the cancer in my breast. If the tests show that the cancer cells might have gone somewhere else, I'll get chemotherapy drugs to kill them wherever they have landed.

"In short," I say, realizing that this is much more than they want, "that's cancer."

"OK," my sons say in unison and leave the kitchen.

The table attached to the nuclear medicine scanner is an ebony plank beneath my hips—rigid and unforgiving. About an hour ago the radioactive tracer was injected into my breast lump, and the nuclear medicine technician began snapping films. Since then he has been watching for the appearance of the tracer in the sentinel node, the lymph node immediately downstream from my cancer. As each successive film is clipped to the view box, I twist my head sideways, eager for an early glimpse of that all-important radioactive node.

For some reason, this examination is being done in the children's hospital nuclear medicine suite rather than in the main hospital. Lying here with the massive, cream-colored scanner looming over me, I feel displaced, in a foreign and yet familiar land. Although I've never been in this room, I have walked the hallways just beyond the door a thousand times, through the corridor that is painted cyanosis—that is, lack of oxygen in the blood—blue and leads from the elevator, past the vending machines, around the corner, to the pediatric radiology reading room. The muffled footfalls outside may belong to my students and colleagues, maybe, even, to the Pediatric Infectious Diseases team making their late morning rounds.

"Hi." It's Jim. Earlier he was at work in the operating room at St. Joseph's Hospital and now has come to University Hospital to be with me.

"It hasn't appeared yet," I say.

We both stare at the view boxes. Each film is a sheet of clear plastic, and along its right edge is a black blob from the tracer that was injected into my tumor. Gazing at x-rays is easy for us, and learning about a new medical procedure, even as participants, is interesting. It draws us back into our comfortable medical world, where cancer is a disease for us to diagnose and to treat but not to have.

As the technician clips another film to the view box, the nuclear medicine physician steps into the room and introduces himself. "Let's take a look," he says, turning to face the row of films. The light from the view box throws an eerie ice blue veil over his forehead, cheeks, nose, chin. His eyes sink into the shadows. He taps the tip of his pen against the most recent film and says, "There it is."

I see it too—a black dot the size of a pinto bean against the transparent plastic of the film. It's lateral to the quarter-sized stain of tracer in the tumor.

"What's that other thing?" I ask. There's a second pinto bean. "The signal medial to the lump?"

"I . . . don't . . . know," he answers, his words stumbling slowly from his mouth.

Obviously it's another node, one in a chain of lymphatics draining medially toward my sternum rather than laterally toward my armpit. The first node to appear on these films lateral to my tumor, the sentinel node, will be removed later this afternoon by my surgeon. What about that medial node? Retrieving it would require cutting through my breast bone, which is too risky an operation for a screening procedure.

I squirm on the rigid scanner table, imagining surgical shears snipping through my sternum to get to that extra node. Myron won't do that, but what if that medial node has cancer in it? We won't know that after the upcoming operation. In fact, we won't know that ever. The image of that second pinto bean, I suspect, will scroll through my head over and over, and I will worry about it for a very long time.

Clearly the nuclear medicine doctor doesn't want to have this conversation about the medial node with me. He can't answer all the questions that would follow. He knows what the medial pinto bean is, but he just doesn't know what, if anything, my surgeon is going to do about it.

Now that the dye has traveled to the sentinel node, my next stop will be the main hospital to check in for my lumpectomy. It's an outpatient procedure. The lump will be removed this afternoon, as will the sentinel node, and I'll go home later in the day to wait for the pathology report on whether my cancer has spread to the node.

As Jim and I gather my things to leave the nuclear medicine suite, the technician says, "Oh, one last thing. Don't be alarmed that your left breast turns blue for a couple days. It'll be from the isosulfan dye." As we walk to the main hospital, I file the image of one blue breast in my mental computer as if it's a Photoshop picture.

In the preanesthesia room rows of cubicles line the walls, a gurney in each cubicle, a patient on each gurney. I'm in the cubicle across from the nurses' station. It's like being a cow, in a stall, in a barn.

Now that I'm settled, rather than thinking of cows, I'm thinking of insects, swarms of them. The nurses, aides, orderlies, and clerks crisscross the floor as if someone kicked the top off an anthill—skittering here, skuttering there. Armed with IV bags, papers, syringes, clipboards, and stacks of linen, they are identical in their uniforms of aqua scrub suits, paper booties, and gauze scrub caps. Some have paper masks hanging from their necks.

It's unnerving here. I don't usually spend much time in operating rooms, and when I do, I'm part of the anthill team rather than the one lying on a gurney, wearing a hospital gown backwards and no underwear. It must be even odder for Jim as a surgeon. We hide behind this morning's *New York Times*, me propped up on the gurney with my reading glasses resting on my nose and Jim seated beside me in a chair.

The *Times'* obituaries are always good reading, and today's paper has a long report of the death of Gene Kelly's brother, also a dancer. It catches my eye because Fred Kelly's niece lives in Ann Arbor. So, while awaiting my lumpectomy, I learn that the Kelly boys were taught to dance by their mother, a vaudeville instructor in Pittsburgh. The article draws my attention away from the scurry all around me.

The anesthesiologist introduces herself and explains that I will be intubated—that an endotracheal tube will be inserted into my windpipe to assure that during the operation I continue to breathe—because 1 to 2 percent of patients have an anaphylactic reaction to the isosulfan dye. That's one in fifty to one in a hundred. I don't remember being told about this potential complication before agreeing to the sentinel node mapping procedure. Too late now.

The nurse inserts an IV into my right hand, connects the tubing that dangles from a bag of clear liquid, and with a flick of her thumb starts the Ringer's lactate flowing. Suddenly my arm is ice cold. I wrap it in the business section of the *Times*, trying to warm up. When the nurse returns and injects my preanesthesia sedatives, I say, "I have a suggestion. Why don't you run the IV bags through the microwave for a few seconds before hooking them up to the patients?"

That's the last thing I remember.

⚘

While I sleep, my cancer and part of the surrounding breast, the golf-ball-size mass of bloody fat and connective tissue newly removed from my body, bumps against the bottom of the specimen bottle during its ride to the pathology laboratory. There the pathologists log the specimen into their database and describe what they see. To the casual observer, it looks like fat from a Butterball turkey, specifically, like the yellowish, greasy gristle immediately behind the plastic twister that holds the ends of the drumsticks together.

The pathology technician measures the specimen. Mine is 6.1 × 3.0 × 7 centimeters (or about 2½ × 1¼ × 2½ inches). Using a scalpel she slices through the mass of tissue and finds a telltale white core that feels gritty, the same sandiness I felt when the needle slid through my tumor during the fine needle aspiration. She measures the distance between the tumor mass and the edges of the lumpectomy specimen, determining whether the surgeon removed enough normal tissue around the tumor to guarantee that none of the cancer was left behind. She describes the nontumor part of the mass, of which 60 percent is fibroglandular tissue—the milk ducts and stringy scaffold supporting the ducts—and 40 percent is adipose, the pathologists' polite word for fat.

The technician then cuts the tumor into very thin wafers, lays them on microscope slides, and stains them with dyes that highlight the structural features of the tissue. A pathologist then studies the stained slices under the microscope and analyzes what she sees. She determines whether the tumor is circumscribed (the cells growing in a tight glob) or invasive (the cells wandering through the tissue, pushing aside the normal structures as they go). She looks for angio-lymphatic invasion, fingers of cancer cells clawing into the walls of blood vessels or lymphatic channels. That's a bad sign, as it signals the setup for metastasis.

Under the microscope, normal cells are orderly. They align themselves into hollow ducts or cluster themselves into milk glands. When they reproduce, they divide into daughter cells just like themselves—same size, same shape, same structural characteristics. On the other hand, cancer cells are messy. They show up where they shouldn't be and display variable physical characteristics—huge cells next to tiny cells, each looking a bit different from its neighbor. In short, cancer is islands of irregular evil among a sea of uniform good.

Breast cancer, however, is not one disease. In fact, just as each human being is different, the biology of each tumor is different. The pathologist distills what she sees in the microscope into one three-word phrase, "invasive ductal carcinoma," knowing that the cancer she has just described—mine—is as different from the last three invasive ductal carcinomas she examined as the women who carry them. Four women. Four different shoe sizes. Four different preferences in soda pop. Four different cancers, all called "invasive ductal carcinoma."

The pathologist wants to know more about my individual cancer, to gauge its special quirks compared to those of other women. My oncologist wants to understand the "warts on its skin," to know as best he can the mysteries it holds deep in its physiology so he can prescribe the best therapy.

Thus, my cancer undergoes further scrutiny. The pathology technician runs it through a gauntlet of tests to describe it more accurately, to ascertain some of its subtle traits that may predict its invasiveness and may dictate certain treatments.

Characterizing my tumor is an exercise in describing particles that fit together. The technician looks for estrogen receptors, molecules on cancer cells that are the "locks" in a biological security system where the "key" is the hormone, estrogen. About 60 percent of breast cancer cells have extra estrogen (E) receptors (R) (i.e., they are ER+) on their

| Reg#: 555555555 | Name: GILSDORF, JANET | DOB: 02/17/1945 | Sex: F | Age: 55 Years |
|---|---|---|---|---|

| ACCN Number | Order Test Code | Order Test Name | Last updated |
|---|---|---|---|
| ACCN: IF-00-0620 | SPF | SP FINAL REPORT | 03-07-2000, 12:58 |
| Collected: 02/25/2000 | | | |

**HISTORY:** A 55-year-old female examined by MD last week found to have left breast mass. Mammogram 2/23/00 revealed a 1.3 cm spiculated mass in left inner, upper quadrant. No associated microcalcifications. Left breast mass, FNA positive 2/23. Left breast lumpectomy with SLN biopsy and ALND.

**GROSS:**

    1. "L breast lumpectomy stitch superior medial" A 6.1 x 3.0 x 7.1 cm fragment of mature-appearing fibroadipose with an attached 3.0 x 1.1 cm ellipse of skin with an attached suture (superior medial). Skin surfaces are previously dyed with blue surgical ink. Deep surface is unremarkable. The lateral half black, the medial green. Sectioning reveals a 2.0 x 1.4 x 1.0 cm white neoplasm with gritty surfaces. The surrounding fibroglandular tissue is previously inked with blue surgical dye. The neoplasm appears to come within 0.2 cm of the green inked (medial) line of resection. The remaining parenchyma is composed of approximately 60% fibroglandular tissue and 40% adipose. See diagram.

1A.-B. Bisected superior tip of skin. (2ss)
1C.-D. Bisected superior-central portion of skin and fibroglandular tissue. (2ss)
1E.-G. Trisected central-inferior ellipse of skin and fibroglandular soft tissue. (3ss)
1H.-I. Superficial portion of inferior half of specimen with lesion closest approximation to black inked (lateral) line of resection.
1J. Inferior half of specimen deep line of resection. (1ss)
2. "True superior margin" Two fragments of fibroadipose, aggregating to 7.0 x 3.5 x 2.0 cm. Inked green.
2A.-C. Soft tissue. (ns)
3. "True inferior margin" A 3.8 x 2.5 x 1.5 cm fragment of mature pink fibroadipose. Entirely submitted in cassette 3A.-C. (ns)
CT

CXT:AMH  03/07/00

**MICROSCOPIC:**
SUMMARY FOR INVASIVE BREAST CARCINOMAS:
- Greatest dimension of invasive carcinoma (micro):  2.0 cm.
- Contour of carcinoma (circumscribed, infiltrative):  Infiltrative.
- Involvement of surgical margins (Pos, Close (< 1 mm), Neg):  Positive (true inferior margin)
- Histopathologic grade (Bloom-Richardson 1-3):  2.
- Lympho-plasmacytic response (Yes, No):  No.
- Peritumoral angio-lymphatic invasion (Yes, No):  Yes.
- Number of lymph nodes with metastases / total number of nodes:  1/3 (cytokeratin stain confirmatory).
- Extranodal soft tissue neoplastic invasion:  No.
- Extensive DCIS (Yes, No):  No.
- DCIS > 25% of tumor (Yes, No):  No.
- Extratumoral DCIS (Yes, No):  Yes.
- Hormonal receptors (Biochemical/Immunohistochemical):  ER,PR positive (by immunohistochemistry).
- Her-2/neu immunohistochemistry is positive for overexpression.

    T1c N1a Mx

**DIAGNOSIS:**
    1.-3. Breast, left, lumpectomy and true superior and inferior margin resections: Invasive ductal carcinoma (2.0 cm, Bloom-Richardson 2) and high grade ductal carcinoma in-situ. Angiolymphatic invasion present. Invasive neoplasm present at "true inferior margin"; all other margins negative for neoplasm.

    Invasive carcinoma positive for estrogen and progesterone receptors as well as overexpression of Her-2/neu (by immunohistochemistry, appropriate controls).

    Please see template. Please see comment.

    John Doe, M.D. / Jane Doe, M.D.

    I, Jane Doe, M.D., the signing staff pathologist, have personally examined and interpreted the slides from this case.

    Code:I

    FC:23207, 23205 (5), 23451 (5)

    "This immunohistochemical stain was developed and its performance characteristics determined by the University of Michigan Clinical Immunoperoxidase Laboratory. It has not been cleared or approved by the U.S. Food and Drug Administration.  (The FDA has determined that such clearance is not necessary. This stain is used for clinical purposes. It should not be regarded as investigational or for research. This laboratory is certified under the Clinical Laboratory Improvement Amendments of 1988 ["CLIA"] as qualified to perform high complexity testing)."

    T04030, P11000, M85003, M80001, M00100, M80103, F26480, F26370, T08000,
    TY8100, P11000, M80106, T04000

    Jane Doe, M.D.
    (electronic signature)

    AFP:AFP:AMH 03/07/00

surfaces, and when they bind to estrogen, the cells undergo a growth spurt. Thus, an estrogen key inserted into the cell's ER lock is akin to fertilizing the thistles. It's interesting that estrogen is stored in fat. Does this make overweight women more feminine? They are definitely more susceptible to breast cancer. Progesterone receptors (PR) are similar to ER, only the key to their locks is progesterone, yet another type of fertilizer for PR+ cancer cells.

The pathologist looks at my cancer for evidence of HER-2/neu, a gene important in cell growth. This gene instructs the cell to make a growth factor that acts as a vitamin for the cell. When breast cancer cells make too much of the growth factor—because there are too many copies of the gene in the cell's chromosome; that is, the gene is over-amplified—the cells rev up and grow faster. This gene has several names (HER-2, neu, HER-2/neu, C-erb B2), and the grim news is that if it's overamplified in my cancer, I will have a poorer prognosis for survival.

The pathologist, in a regimented series of observations, describes what she sees on my specimen and issues her report.

This is my cancer, the way it looks, the way it's eating its way into my tissues.

In the meanwhile I sleep, nestled in the never-never land of weird, anesthesia-induced oblivion, protected from the reality that unfolds around me. The pathologists and my surgeons and anesthesiologists and nurses are doing their jobs while I'm doing mine—living and being and dreaming and giving up a part of me, my cancer.

# CHAPTER 7

### *The Nodes Know*

*A voice echoes through a tunnel* as if bouncing off the walls of a long, narrow space. Maybe it's a yard in length, maybe a mile. The words undulate as if spoken underwater and then tumble together like poured wine. Someone touches my right elbow, lifts it away from my body. The fingers are warm. The sound of fabric being torn rustles near my ear. My right arm is growing, inflating, filling with air. Tight. Tighter. Tighter yet.

The voice speaks again. This time I understand. "Blood pressure, hon . . ." Her words are cut short by the rip of Velcro.

I try to open one eye. The light is blinding so I clamp it shut again.

"Do you have to use the bathroom?" she asks.

"No," I mumble. Why is she asking these questions? Who is she? Where am I?

My throat burns. Through both eyes, now, I squint against the bright glare. A curtain of aqua and peach stripes hangs before me.

"Are you awake?" It's Jim, on my left.

"Don't know."

"Your operation is over." His fingers, rough from years of surgical soap and scrub brushes, stroke my forehead. I can smell that he is near me, can sense his familiar, spicy scent of cinnamon and mangoes.

Later—an hour, a year—the nurse asks, "Ready for the bathroom yet?"

"Yes." The IV bag is empty and my bladder is full.

"How about walking?" She hooks up a new bag of IV fluid.

"Where is it?"

She waves her arm toward the far corner of this huge room.

"Where?"

She points to a distant door.

"I'll be a heap on the floor before I'm halfway there."

"OK, we'll get you a ride." The shrug of her shoulders suggests I'm being a giver-upper or maybe a pest.

She returns, pushing a wheelchair. With Jim's help, she moves me to the seat and hangs the new IV bag on the chair's pole.

Even later, the nurse lays my discharge papers on the sheet that covers my legs. "Dr. Gilsdorf, you're free to go."

My throat aches. Waves of nausea float like bilious green vapor through me. My arms are so weak I couldn't lift a paperclip. "Jim, I need more sleep."

"You can sleep when we get home."

The room is quiet, the scurrying people are gone. The curtains that separate the cubicles are drawn back against the wall. On each gurney rests a neatly folded gown atop a neatly folded sheet atop a neatly folded plastic clothes sack atop a neatly folded flannel blanket. I'm the last patient here.

Jim and the nurse load me into the wheelchair again.

"Where's the car?" I ask.

"In the parking garage." Jim wraps a flannel blanket around my shoulders. "Where's your coat?"

"In my office. We'll have to stop there on the way to the car."

He pushes the wheelchair out the surgical suite door. The floor of the hallway is freshly waxed. It shines like satin.

Waves of nausea continue to lick my face. I'm dizzy. I'm shedding cold sweat. My right elbow rests on the arm of the wheelchair, and my right hand cradles my head. The corridor that leads, eventually, to my office is just ahead.

"Jim, skip the coat. Take me to the car."

"It's February, Janet, and cold outside."

"I don't care. I have to get back to bed as soon as possible."

Jim helps me into his van. My breath turns to smoke in the frigid air. The front seat feels like a block of ice. He wraps a second flannel blanket, the one that pads the wheelchair seat, around my shoulders.

"I'll be back in a minute," he says, stepping away from the van.

"Where're you going?"

"To take the wheelchair back."

"No you're not. Leave it here. If they can't escort us to the car, they can figure out how to retrieve the chair. I have to go home." Thank God we live only a couple miles away, or I don't think I could make it.

❧

It's been almost twenty-four hours since my operation, and I feel as if I've been run over by a fully loaded moving van.

"Jim, what did they do to me?" I try to roll over. "Let me fall off the operating room table or something? I ache everywhere. Even my ears ache."

"You were intubated. Remember? The succinylcholine they used to paralyze you depolarized all the nerve endings in your body. Every muscle you own was drained of its electrical energy."

"Feels like it still is."

Intubated. A tube stuffed down my windpipe. That explains why my throat still hurts. It feels as if the tube was wrapped in barbed wire.

In the afternoon Bean, my daughter-in-law, leans against the door frame into our bedroom. She's a trim, dainty woman with shiny hair the color of raisins. She fits into my son Daniel's life like a dollar in a wallet. With enormous grace, she brings out the best in him, gives purpose to his being, laughs at his antics. Yet, she sticks up for herself. She scolds him (privately) when he does something thoughtless. She puts a cautious lid on his risk-taking ways. Together they settle on weird, interesting choices in their lifestyle. Amazingly, they agree on the chickens in the backyard of their Portland home, on the orange paint on the dining room walls, on the wood-burning stove instead of a functional furnace.

Bean asks, "Where do you keep the silver polish?"

Grunts and giggles drift in from the living room. My sons are arm wrestling, the younger one in a lifelong quest to best his big brother, the older one sure to win because he's six feet, four inches tall.

"Under the kitchen sink. Why?"

"You'll see."

Minutes later she returns, carrying a tray with warm soup in a china bowl, a cloth napkin, a sterling spoon, and water in a wineglass. She smooths my quilt and arranges the tray on my lap. The soup smells of curry. Little islands of potato and onion bob in its creamy liquid.

While sons are wonderful, daughters, including daughters-in-law, are gifts beyond value. Besides feeding me, Bean sends Dan to the bookstore for the *New York Times*, since it can't, for some inexplicable reason, be delivered to our address. Furthermore, she toted, all the way from Oregon, past issues of *Threads* magazine for me to read.

She sets my silver bell, a previously tarnished but now sparkling North Dakota centennial souvenir, on my bedside cabinet.

"If you need anything, just ring," she says. With a bow, she exits the bedroom.

After a few minutes, I pick up the bell. "DING. DING. DING."

Bean races from the hallway to my side. "What do you need?"

"Nothing." I smile. "This is a test, to be sure the system works."

She laughs and shakes her head as she returns to the kitchen.

The next morning Jim helps me remove the dressings from my chest so I can take a shower. My fingers shake as I claw at the bandages. What will my chest look like? Will I have a recognizable breast after they carved out the lump? Can I live with it for the rest of my life?

Off comes the paper and elastic bandeau with its Velcro closure. Off come the four-by-four-inch gauze squares that are stained with wound ooze. My cancer is gone. It now rests in a freezer in the pathology laboratory. All that remains in me are the memories and the incisions. I raise my left arm to shed the dressings and a searing pain stabs through my chest.

I look down. There it is, my new breast. The slightly red, slightly raised two-inch gooey line of the lumpectomy incision runs above my left nipple. Another two-inch cut, where the sentinel nodes were removed, rides the fold of my left armpit.

It isn't so bad. The swelling will go down with time, and I'll have a somewhat, but not hideously, distorted breast.

The next week, Jim accompanies me to the post–lumpectomy/sentinel node biopsy clinic visit. We're about to learn whether the sentinel node that Myron removed is positive or negative, whether my cancer has spread beyond the almond that used to be in my breast. As we wait, Jim's left knee jumps seemingly in synchrony with his heartbeat. He picks at a grease spot on his pants leg. Although his right shoulder is only eight inches from my left shoulder, he seems at least twelve light-years away. He doesn't want to be here, doesn't want to hear the news from the surgeon if it's bad, doesn't want to face the possibility that it could, indeed, *be* bad. As a general surgeon, Jim does a lot of "breast work" and thus spends many hours of every day on the other side—the medical side—of the brick wall that looms tall and broad between doctors and patients. He doesn't like being on this side—the wrong side, the helpless side—of that wall. Neither do I.

The examining room door swings wide, and my surgeon, a welcoming smile slashed across his face, walks in. "Hi, Jim," he says, offering my husband his hand. "How's it going?"

"I've been better," Jim responds, shaking Myron's hand.

Myron nods, turns toward me. "Well, we have the report." He glances at the printed page in his hand and wastes no more time getting to the point. He's handling this just as I want him to: matter of factly, no pirouetting around the truth.

"Your cancer is a grade II ductal carcinoma. It's ER/PR positive and HER2/neu positive."

To me right now, these details of my cancer are like a description of the inside of my stomach. I can't see it, have never seen one in living color, can't imagine what it looks or smells like. I can't relate to his words as anything other than a distant string of sounds. I can't process this information clearly today, and these terms seem like a med school exam question that doesn't pertain to me. They are, however, etched in my mind so that I can retrieve them later and hopefully, then, sort them out and find their ultimate meaning.

"As you know," Myron continues, "we harvested three nodes in the sentinel node dissection." I wince at the word *harvested*. It's an unfortunate word that is common jargon among doctors and best not overheard by patients. It doesn't alarm me. I, too, use it in speaking to my colleagues, but I've never heard it from this vantage point before.

"Two of the nodes are negative." He pauses, stares squarely into my eyes, and takes a breath. "One is positive."

Jim utters a groan and grabs my hand.

"The pathologist noted some angio-lymphatic invasion in your tumor," Myron adds.

A reel of blurry cartoons spools through my mind. ER/PR positive. I see sinister-looking cells decorated with knobs and baubles to which velvety estrogen and progesterone molecules dock. Angio-lymphatic invasion. I see cells sporting deep purple nucleoli meandering into the walls of my blood vessels. Like an ugly oil spill, they ooze between normal cells, relentlessly forging uncharted trails into my healthy tissues.

As the colorful pictures of my tumor fade, my mind instantly begins calculating the course ahead: axillary dissection, chemotherapy for sure. The positive node, indicating that the tumor has spread beyond my breast, and the angio-lymphatic invasion mean a worse prognosis, which dictates more intensive treatment.

My little dalliance with cancer just turned into a very serious deal. I was counting on a "touch" of malignancy that the lumpectomy and radiation would cure. Nothing more. Not this. Deep inside my chest, beneath my healing lumpectomy incision, my heart bangs against my ribs. My stomach sinks into my shoes. Someone has tied a rope around my chest and I can't breath. My hands clutch Jim's.

"The pathologists can't be sure that the margins are clean," Myron adds. The rope around my lungs tightens. That means another operation to excise more breast tissue from the previous operative bed.

As if Myron and I are engaged in a peculiar dance, he steps right in and says, "So, when we do the axillary dissection, we'll also excise more tissue around the lumpectomy bed."

The examining room door bangs behind Myron as he leaves. Jim shakes his head violently as if he's been bit on the ear by a bee. A roar of expletives explodes from him.

I should be used to this savage response. Every time he makes a wrong cut in a block of wood with his table saw, or sands a surface too deep, or steps on a sharp doggy toy in his stocking feet, he utters the same expletives. But I hate it and will never get used to it. I want to smother the outbursts before they begin, to exterminate their cause, fix the problem, make it pretty. At least I want, somehow, for the magnitude of his response to be proportional to the problem. Whenever I hear the expletives rising over the whir of the saw blade from the basement, I imagine his severed hand lying among the wood shavings on the floor.

But, then, maybe he got it right today. Maybe hearing that the cancer has spread to his wife's lymph nodes justifies every profane word he can think of. I just don't want to be around to hear it.

What's *my* reaction to my surgeon's news? Mostly I'm numb—taking in the facts, rearranging the upcoming commitments that litter the next year of my life. What will I do about my clinical responsibilities? Will I be able to attend Joe's graduation in Monterey, California? The family reunion in North Dakota? What about the talk I agreed to give to the Interscience Conference on Antimicrobial Agents and Chemotherapeutics in Toronto? Should I take the Pediatric Infectious Diseases recertification exam in May? I'm registered and all paid up. And I'm supposed to fly to Philadelphia in two weeks for a meeting of the committee that writes questions for the National Board of Medical Examiners. The questions I was assigned, all one hundred of them, are written. Will I be able to make the trip? My appointment calendar flies through my head, and a mental eraser now transforms each page into a blank sheet.

I'll do what I can at work. I can't imagine not completing the projects I have begun, not fulfilling the professional responsibilities that define who I am, that frame my life. I have a research laboratory to direct, two NIH grants to oversee, the Pediatric Infectious Diseases division to lead. I have students to train and patients who depend on me for their medical care. I can't just disappear and leave them all dangling.

After hearing my surgeon's words, I'm also preparing myself for another operation, two big incisions this time—the axillary dissection cut and the redo of the lumpectomy. I'm preparing for another anesthetic and for chemotherapy. The row of formerly upright, evenly spaced, well-controlled dominos—plans, expectations, hopes for the upcoming year, for the rest of my life—are now collapsing one after the other, led by that positive node.

The reality of the news hangs in the stuffy examining room air. It's a swarming miasma now at arm's length from me; it soon ventures close and then swirls away again. I'm safe in a padded space of normality, secure and bolstered by denial. This isn't really happening. It's a B movie, a sappy novel, a terrible mistake.

The next day, I boot up my computer at home and log into the laboratory database that is accessible only to university doctors—and nurses and clerks and students and anyone else who has a password—and read the report of my lymph nodes.

| Reg#: 555555555 | Name: GILSDORF, JANET | | DOB: 02/17/1945 | Sex: F | Age: 55 Years |
|---|---|---|---|---|---|
| **ACCN Number** | | **Order Test Code** | **Order Test Name** | | **Last updated** |
| ACCN: IF-00-0620 | | SPF | SP FINAL REPORT | | 03-07-2000, 12:58 |
| Collected: 02/25/2000 | | | | | |

**GROSS:** 1. "Warm nodes blue L axilla" Three fragments of mature-appearing fibroadipose, 2.3 x 2.5 x 1.0 cm. Entirely submitted in cassettes 4A.-B. (ns)
    2. "Hot blue node #1 L axilla" A 2.0 x 1.4 x 1.4 cm piece of mature-appearing fibroadipose containing a palpable lymph node. Bisected and entirely submitted in cassettes 5A.-B. (ns)
    3. "Very hot blue node L axilla" A 2.6 x 1.5 x 1.5 cm piece of mature-appearing fibroadipose containing a palpable probable lymph node. Bisected and entirely submitted in cassettes 6A.-B.

**MICROSCOPIC:**
SUMMARY FOR INVASIVE BREAST CARCINOMA
    1. Lymph node, left axilla, warm blue, excision: One lymph node negative for neoplasm.
    2. Lymph node, left axilla, hot blue #1, excision: One lymph node negative for neoplasm, cytokeratin stain by immunohistochemistry confirmatory.
    3. Lymph node, left axilla, very hot blue, excision: One lymph node positive for metastatic carcinoma.

Checking my own lab results isn't illegal or immoral or forbidden by patient confidentiality rules. Until now, I haven't done that, haven't wanted to get my medical information over cyberspace. I wanted to hear it, in person, from Myron; to hear the inflection of his voice, the tempo of the pauses in his speech; to see the angle of his eyes, the tilt of his head. That's how I know what the information really means.

I print the report and hand it to Jim. He glances briefly at the page and sets it on the stack of magazines beside his La-Z-Boy. Myron relayed very adequately the important message from the report. For Jim, the spoken details sting too much. He doesn't need to read them, too.

# Chapter 8

*Interlude. Adrift.*

*Now I wait.* My lumpectomy and sentinel node biopsy incisions need to heal before Myron can do the next operation, the lumpectomy revision to remove possible residual tumor and the axillary dissection to remove the nodes from my armpit so they can be examined for metastatic cancer. It might seem like an odd concept—letting the incisions knit together so they can be torn apart again. But vibrant, injured tissue mends better than sick, injured tissue.

The waiting is time at a near standstill, inching forward with neck bent, head down, eyes riveted to the ground. Our children have returned to their homes far away—Dan and Bean to Oregon and Joe to California, leaving a hole I can't fill. Today's empty minutes are carried into tomorrow, one slow second at a time.

While waiting, I continue to work, but less efficiently than before. Cancer has proven to be heavy. It's like hauling a sack of rocks uphill. My thoughts are empty—not anguished, not terrified, not furious, just empty. I read each paragraph in biomedical journals three times and still don't know what was written. I open files on my computer and don't recall what I wanted from them. I can't remember the exact details of my patients' illnesses and have to review their case summaries before answering phone calls.

At home, I still cook and knit. To occupy the sluggish hours, I have begun to play solitaire. In the evening after I've read the newspaper, I prop the kidney-shaped lapboard Jim made for me across the arms of my easy chair and deal out the cards. It keeps my hands busy and my mind distracted. Just as cream neutralizes the bitter in the coffee, solitaire neutralizes the unease in my head.

I'm getting pretty good at the six cards up, once through the deck version I learned as a child. It's a game of opportunity. The secret to winning is to keep all options open, to make no unnecessary moves, and to release aces early. This game requires concentration and discipline—good antidotes to worry. About a quarter of the time I win. Sometimes, rarely, I win two in a row. Other times, especially on the bad days, I play for up to an hour, losing game after game after game.

My healing surgical wounds don't hurt exactly. They don't even ache, at least not in the usual way. Yet, they're pulsating evidence that I have cancer. Whenever I flip a page of the newspaper, wipe a dish, fold the laundry, turn the steering wheel, reach for the phone, or type an e-mail message, the memory of my cancer, escorted by the zing through my left arm, blows apart the placid, painless, fairytale place where I have always lived. Like a nagging mother, my healing incisions are pick-pick-picky and relentless. They mold my future, are an ever-present reminder that my choices aren't infinite anymore, that, in fact, they have dwindled to an unappealing few.

At the bookstore I select a spiral-bound notebook. A collage of dried leaves and torn sheet music decorates its cover. The pages inside are blank. This will be my journal, my cancer journal. Since this ordeal is going to be more complicated than I originally planned, I need to keep track of my thoughts in a classier way than my regular journal, the five-by-eight legal pad.

Jim and I wait in an examining room in the Cancer Center again, this time for the introductory visit with my oncologist. I know Ben, like the rest of my doctors, from medical school committees. But I don't know him well. That makes it easier for me to be his patient.

A large man, he bursts into the room, introduces himself to Jim, and sits down on the examining stool. Paddling his feet against the carpet, he rolls the stool into the space immediately in front of us. It's a gesture of caring, of being available. It signals a willingness to be close to us. The wrinkles beside his eyes tell of kindness.

He reviews my medical history, reviews the pathology findings from my tumor. Then he examines me. There's magic in his touch. Through his warm hands, the liqueur of respect—reassuring and reaffirming, soothing and therapeutic—moves like a lullaby from him to me.

Providing medical care for another physician is sometimes a doctor's worst nightmare. Physicians can be terrible patients, argumentative, distrustful, demanding, poorly compliant. They ask a million questions, try to take shortcuts, want to exercise veto power over every aspect of their care. In short, physician-patients can't quit being the physician.

I clarify the rules. "I'm the patient, you're the doctor. I won't try to second-guess your medical decisions."

"Good," he nods. "That's a deal."

He begins to explain what I can expect from the chemotherapy: the dosing schedule, the side effects, the attendant precautions. "You'll receive four doses of Adriamycin and Cytoxan and then possibly a course of Taxol. We'll decide about that after I return from an upcoming clinical oncology meeting."

He reminds me that my risk of infection will be high because my white blood cells will be low. "Do you do any gardening?" he asks, turning over my left hand, running his fingers along my left forearm.

"Yes."

"Always wear gloves and long sleeves. We don't want you to get injured and infected on that left hand or arm. If you do, at the very first sign of an infection, start taking Cipro. Start it immediately and then call me."

He estimates the impact of the therapy on my life. "You'll be able to work if you want to, Janet, but not sixty hours a week."

How does he know my usual schedule? How does he know that I'm sometimes at my desk until eight o'clock at night, that I rarely get home before seven, that I catch up on my medical reading in the evening and on the weekends, that I haul satchels of work on vacation? He knows because, at the university, we all overdo it.

"You'll be more fatigued than usual." He pauses a moment. When he begins speaking again, his words are emphatic. "You have to understand that your hair *will fall out*," he says, patting my hand.

Earlier in this visit I promised Ben I wouldn't second-guess his medical decisions—and I fully intend to keep that promise—but I don't live in medical isolation. I've subscribed, along with other scientific publications, to the *New England Journal of Medicine* since my medical student days. Previously I would have ignored cancer articles in favor of those about infectious diseases. Now, of course, I study the cancer articles carefully.

"I saw the piece in this week's *New England Journal* about monitoring bone marrow tumor markers to assess metastatic spread of breast cancer," I say, offhandedly.

He stares sternly at me, parsing my words. Experienced physician that he is, he knows the unspoken question behind my comment, which is "Why aren't you using this new technique on me?"

"That study doesn't pertain to you," he says. He takes a deep breath. "Think about it a minute." He then explains the true meaning of the article.

Makes sense. That's why he's the cancer doctor. He knows these things.

In the car on the way home, Jim says, "I like that guy. I *really* like that guy."

My friend Claire, another physician, takes me to lunch. March in Michigan is usually overcast, muddy, and miserable, but today the sun shines through the bare branches of the trees and the warm, clean air offers the promise, even if it's a tease, of spring. Our boots kick the slushy snow as we walk away from our offices, away from the medical campus, away from our work, toward the restaurants in Ann Arbor's Kerrytown district.

The wood-framed houses that line Ann Street have stood there for over a century. Some are probably older than any person currently alive in Ann Arbor. They have endured many winters, withstood many storms. Over the years these stately buildings that once housed families of the faculty have been carved into apartments, home to generations of energetic, idealistic, messy university students. Their porches now sag under the weight of snow-soaked couches and broken tables. Cigarette butts and candy wrappers and gloves without mates, their fingers frozen in grotesque configurations, litter the yards.

"Where will you get your treatment?" Claire asks.

"Cancer Center."

"Our cancer center?"

"Sure," I say.

"Why?"

"Why not?" I ask in return. The thought of receiving my treatment at another institution hasn't occurred to me.

She is, of course, considering where she would get treatment if she were ill. She's thinking of the legions of hospital employees who would have access to her medical records. The University Health System's patient information database supposedly monitors its users, thus assuring confidentiality. None of us trust that. If I were being treated for a sexually transmitted disease or substance abuse or domestic assault, I might be more nervous about exposure. But breast cancer is hardly scandalous, and my past medical history, social history, and family history make for very boring reading.

She's also thinking of loss of dignity and loss of control and of the public nature of these losses if she were treated in her own community. She's thinking humiliation. I'm sure she would seek medical care elsewhere if she were in my situation. Leaving her home, her friends, her routines, her husband for months on end might not bother her, but it's unthinkable for me.

"I'm very comfortable getting my treatment here," I say. "Where do you think I should go? Memorial Sloan-Kettering? M. D. Anderson? Mayo?"

"Oh, I don't know." She appears aware of my defensiveness.

As we walk, I think of how common breast cancer is. Many doctors have a lot of experience with it. Treatment guidelines authored by expert panels of cancer surgeons, oncologists, and radiation oncologists are widely available and used by most physicians who treat patients with breast cancer.

Would I get better medical care at Big Name Cancer Hospital (as if our cancer center isn't big name enough!)? No. Good medicine is, after all, a range of activities rather than one, and only one, acceptable practice. The variation in acceptable practices allows for the patients' unique, individual situations. As Cinderella's ugly stepsisters learned, "one size fits all" doesn't work. That would be a very bad way to treat someone with cancer.

Couldn't I get the newest drugs at Big Name Cancer Hospital? Yes. Experimental therapies are available at any large cancer center, certainly at ours, but I don't need them. While standard treatment doesn't guarantee cure, neither do experimental treatments. If I were failing standard therapy or had a very rare tumor, maybe I'd consider opting for clinical trial protocols. Maybe. Then I would have to decide where I could get the most reasonable ones.

Furthermore, I don't want to travel for my treatment. Airplanes and airports are horrible under the best of circumstances and unspeakable when you're sick. Living out of a hotel room, no matter how luxurious, while receiving cancer therapy would be unimaginably lonely.

Claire and I are a block from our destination, Zingerman's Delicatessen. The sun has ducked behind a shelf of clouds, the leading edge of a gray front that stretches to the western horizon.

"What percentage of your time do you think about having cancer?" she asks.

I'm stunned at the question, have to think awhile for the answer. Claire is brilliant and insightful and blunt.

"About 85 to 90 percent," I finally say.

Hot water from the dispenser at my office runs in an even drizzle over the used tea bag that lies limp in the bottom of my cup. I'm hopeful that another warm drink will tame my thinking. I'm trying to edit a paper written by my postdoctoral student, but my thoughts won't stay with the manuscript. Rather, my mind dances among the myriad facts I have learned about breast cancer. I check my e-mail—delete a few, answer a few, save a few for another time. I stare out the dusty window at the driveway to the children's hospital. I pick the bagel crumbs from between the buttons of my computer's keyboard. Even after the latest cup of tea, I can't concentrate.

As I think about my upcoming surgery and chemotherapy, I realize I'm confused. If I'm going to have chemo drugs to kill every cancer cell lurking in my body, what is the axillary node dissection for? We already know my cancer has spread beyond my breast. I make yet another cup of tea, using a fresh bag this time, and send an e-mail to my oncologist.

From: Janet Gilsdorf
To: oncdoctor@umich.edu
Date: March 10, 2000 9:48:07 AM
Subject: Question
Ben,
Somehow I missed an important concept—why am I having the axillary node dissection? Is it for staging purposes? Does the degree of axillary involvement dictate the intensity or type of chemo? Or is it simply to debulk the tumor?
Janet

From: Benjamin Miller
To: janetgils@umich.edu
Date: March 11, 2000 10:27:32 AM
Subject: Re: Question
The intensity of therapy does depend on the extent of nodal involvement. By removing the lateral nodes, the xrt portals can be limited. I wouldn't want your brachial plexus to become fibrotic.
Ben

From: Janet Gilsdorf
To: oncdoctor@umich.edu
Date: March 10, 2000 11:03:28 AM
Subject: Re: Re: Question
Ben,
Neither would I. Thanks.
Janet

So, the results of the axillary dissection will dictate, to some extent, my treatment. Also, since the lateral nodes will be surgically removed, they won't have to be included in the radiation therapy field. Irradiating the brachial nerves, which are in the same region as the lateral nodes, might result in scars that trap the major nerve to my arm. Now I understand.

My next project rests in the catalogs stacked on the hassock beside my easy chair. I pick the one on top, from Talbots, and begin turning the pages. Since I'm going to have a big operation and then months of chemo, I will do a lot of lounging. I need lounging clothes.

I have no slacks or pants of any kind. For years I have worn only skirts that reach to my ankles: to work, to the grocery store, in the garden, even when canoeing. I think I look terrible in pants so I hide my lumpy figure under yards of billowing fabric. In the evenings, between work and bed, I wear ratty gray sweatpants that belonged to one of my sons and an old flannel shirt.

While recovering from my next operation, I don't want to lie around in my nightgown or those rump-sprung sweatpants. I want to maintain a rhythm to my days, want to get up, get dressed, have a life, get undressed, go to bed. That's what a new cancer wardrobe will do—motivate me to put on clothes.

A velour, two-piece outfit in the Coldwater Creek catalog catches my eye. It's a pretty color, slate blue. The pants are loose with elastic at the waist. The top has buttons so I can get it on after the axillary dissection.

Last night Jim went with me to the Briarwood Mall. I tried on three sets of pants and tops and hated them all. Then I became overwhelmed and discouraged and mad. Too many people, too much noise, too many options. Catalog shopping is much better.

I end up ordering several outfits. An olive green linen jacket and loose pants. A black and white checkered top and black stretch pants. And the slate blue velour.

My writerly friend Emmy says that my new wardrobe, easy-going, comfortable, relaxed, is a good metaphor for life after cancer. Nice idea. Hope it's true.

Jane has cut my hair for over twenty years. We have an agreement—when I'm rich and famous she will travel with me as my personal hairdresser. When she's rich and famous, I will accompany her as her personal physician. Never mind that I'm a pediatrician and she's nearing fifty years old.

I settle into Jane's salon chair, and she snaps the cape around my neck. As she parts my hair and begins to clip, I tell her that I have breast cancer. She pulls the comb and scissors back against her body and says, "Oh, Janet." Her face twists with anguish. "That's awful."

"What do you know about wigs?" I ask.

"Lots." She begins clipping again. "Call me when you're ready and I'll go wig shopping with you. We'll find something nice."

As she finishes my haircut we agree that when it starts to fall out, she will see me immediately to cut it very short. I read about that strategy somewhere. Seems like a better idea than dealing with long threads of loose hair.

Chris Coyle, our son Dan's friend—formerly passing through Boulder, Colorado, where Dan went to college, and presently passing through Portland, Oregon, where Dan lives—calls.

"Louie [one of the artists in Daniel's tattoo shop in Portland] told me about your illness, Mrs. Gilsdorf. I decided to extend my best wishes by phone."

Chris's call is a surprise. I've met him only a few times while he was freeloading a spot on Daniel's sofa in Boulder and monopolizing the TV. The story, which fits into the "pile of hogwash" category of information, was that Chris needed to watch a lot of television because he suffers from attention deficit disorder.

"Louie says they got it all, so that's good." Chris is trying, I'm sure, to convince himself.

I don't tell him that, actually, they didn't "get it all," at least not the first time, that the margins of the original lumpectomy looked as if they still contained tumor cells. Furthermore, there's no way to know whether metastases have already riddled my brain, bones, lungs, or liver. I don't tell him that, either. He's trying to be hopeful.

"Mrs. Gilsdorf, I'm really glad they caught it early."

I also don't explain the naïveté of the *catching it early* notion. In cancer, earlier is always better than later, but in breast cancer, a tumor can be present for only a short time—maybe *caught early*—and, yet, have spawned distant metastases. Likewise, some large tumors— maybe *caught later*—may never spread beyond the breast. So, *early* and *late* have limited meaning in the prognosis of breast cancer.

Chris is saying that he wants me, his friend's mom, to be well. He wants to believe that I'm cured. *Early* and *got it all* are, after all, code words for *cured*. He isn't comfortable, however, using the word *cured* because the opposite of that is *not cured*, just as the opposite of *curable* is *not curable*, and no one wants to wander into those concepts when speaking directly to a cancer patient.

"Good luck, Mrs. Gilsdorf," Chris says. "I might not see you on your next trip to Oregon, because I'm heading to work at a snowboarding camp in Utah."

I'm very moved by his call and amazed at his courage and thoughtfulness in making it.

※

The radiation therapy suite is in the cellar of the hospital, underground, I suppose, so that errant radioactive rays will scatter into the dirt rather than into people on the level below. The waiting room, though, is like a walk-out basement, with windows and a door to a parking lot carved into the hill that slopes down to the river. The rest of the suite, windowless and claustrophobic, burrows into the ground beneath the main hospital.

This is my first appointment with my radiation oncologist. It's an introductory meeting, as my radiation therapy won't begin for months. As with all my doctors, I know Jackie from medical school committees.

My hospital gown is on backwards, the standard breast cancer style, with two ties in the front that fail to keep the edges together. The fabric is thin, easy for the doctor to push aside. The ties are few, easy for the doctor to quickly undo. The garment is short, easy on the hospital's budget. My clothes are stacked in a tight little pile on the chair. My underwear, today the color of eggplants, is discretely folded beneath my sweater. I perch on the end of the examining table and open the pediatric journal I have brought. Even without underwear I want to seem busy. I want to be busy.

There's a knock at the door, and Jackie enters. Wearing a white clinical coat, she strides over to me, wraps her arms around my shoulders, pats my back, moves away, stares into the deepest regions of my eyes, and says, "I'm so very, very sorry you have to go through this."

I drink in her kindness, her gentleness, her empathy. She'll be with me on this journey, will help me find the way along the obscure, hidden path.

The silk flowers at Frank's Nursery and Crafts are arranged by color. Baskets crowded with blooms line the aisles: white dogwood blossoms, cream rosebuds, ivory blowsy peonies, as well as pink dogwood blossoms, crimson rosebuds, and burgundy blowsy peonies. Over the past two weeks I have ordered three wide-brimmed straw hats. Now I need flowers for the hats.

I choose several. Then several more. And yet more. By the time I leave the store, I have two huge plastic sacks full of silk flowers.

They're not real, but they're beautiful, brightly colored, and delicately shaped. They make me think of spring, of summer, of warm weather, of comfort, of growing things, of freshness, of the lilacs and irises and lilies in our yard. They won't wilt, won't turn to gray, dry nubbins at the end of their time. They are merely a stand-in for real flowers, of course, but right now artificial blooms are the best I can do.

I write in my journal:

> *It's like being in a play—repeating the same stories over and over, rehearsing the words and pauses and effects. My new reality is a character role, a cancer patient, and I walk in her footprints, speak her words, perform her actions. According to the script, I, the actress, arrange for a wig, reorganize work activities, provide telephone updates to friends and relatives, cancel the trip to the National Board in Philadelphia, cancel the Pediatric Infectious Diseases recertifying examination.*
>
> *The new role isn't a perfect fit for the real me. It takes work to learn the lines, to walk the walk. And at the end of the day, I can't remove the costume, or wipe away the makeup, or stow the affectations of the character in a drawer. At the end of the day, the character is me and the role is my new identity.*

# Chapter 9

*Pain and Mutilation*

*I'm back on a gurney, in a cubicle,* in the preanesthesia room, reading the *New York Times*. The comings and goings of the operating room personnel don't interest me. Nothing of the surgical experience is new anymore. Rather than intriguing, now it's dark and oppressive. The novelty of having cancer, small as it was, has completely disappeared.

A surgery resident approaches with the informed consent document. This young doctor attended medical school at the university, was an officer in Alpha Omega Alpha, the medical honor society. I first met him at an AΩA dinner. He seems embarrassed to see me here, doesn't know how to approach a professor who is dressed in a hospital gown, lying on a gurney.

"Ah, Doctor Gilsdorf," he stutters. "We need to have the consent signed." His eyes trail off to the side. He hands me the papers as if they are toxic.

I don't need to read them. I know what they say: date, name of patient, name of surgeon, type of operation, list of possible complications. They say that I acknowledge that the operation may need to be extended due to unforeseen circumstances, that anesthesia poses potential adverse events, that there is no promise of successful outcome, that transfusions offer risks and benefits, that trainees may be involved in my care, that I give permission for the hospital to dispose of all removed tissue. With the resident's pen, I write my name on the line labeled *Patient Signature*.

The anesthesiologist, a woman Jim knows well, explains that I won't be intubated for this procedure. Rather, they'll use a new type of oral airway to keep me breathing during my operation. Truth be told,

I'm terrified of anesthesia. At the Indian Health Service hospital in Owyhee, Nevada, where we worked to fulfill Jim's military obligation during the Vietnam War, a middle-aged woman named Agnes lived out her long life functioning as a four-month-old, the result of anesthesia gone bad during a routine gall bladder operation. I like to be in control of things that are important, and breathing is as important as it gets. Shortly I'll be totally dependent on a stranger for my breathing. Should I trust the system to take care of me while I'm unconscious? I know things sometimes go awry. What choices do I have? Axillary dissection without anesthesia? No way! I hope they know what they're doing.

The nurse injects the sedative into my IV. I'm groggy, but awake, during the ride into the surgical suite. There, the huge, bright eye of the OR light stares down at me.

"Can you slide over to the table?" someone asks.

Several hands, confident and strong, support my body as I slide from the gurney to the operating table. That's the last thing I remember.

Every surgical procedure is a violation of a person's integrity, an opening up of places that never before have seen a beam of light or felt the stir of air. After my left armpit is swabbed with disinfectant and then draped in sterile towels and sheets so as to leave a peek hole to my body, my surgeon slices through my skin. With a sharp scalpel blade, he makes elliptical incisions, two swift parentheses, that encompass my previous sentinel node biopsy scar. Then, with gloved fingers he separates the muscles and pushes them to the side, exposing the underlying tissues in which my axillary lymph nodes reside. My body parts—the axillary vein, pectoralis minor muscle, latissimus dorsi muscle, and the junction of the latissimus and serratus muscles—are the landmarks that guide him to the correct space. From this anatomic box he removes a bloody softball-sized clump of fat that contains the lymph nodes. He's careful to avoid injuring the long thoracic nerve and the thoracodorsal neurovascular bundle. In order to remove all the nodes, however, he has to cut through the intercostobrachial nerve.

After completing the axillary dissection, the surgical team members change gowns, gloves, and instruments to avoid contaminating the new surgical site with possible tumor cells. They then proceed to enlarge my former lumpectomy bed.

Hard as Myron tries to avoid damage to the healthy tissue, unintended and often unpreventable consequences occur. Arteries and veins are nicked and blood oozes. Muscles are compressed and nerves are stretched, crushed, or severed. In the end, the cancerous lump and lymph nodes are gone, and I'm left with two deep, ragged holes.

Riding the dawn of anesthesia withdrawal, I awaken in slow motion. Light glimmers. I'm cold. It's quiet. I'm alone. The smell is medicinal. Wheels rumble in the distance, a faint, echolike clickity-clack. Walls surround me. A window. A door.

Through one open eye I glance out the window. I'm in a "court-side" room, one facing the little park surrounded by medical center buildings. The other option would be a "riverside" room. This is fine. I certainly don't care what kind of room I have.

The windows in University Hospital are set lower on the walls than in many buildings so patients can see the outside world from their beds. On the grounds of the courtyard, someone has stomped "HELLO PAT" into the snow. Who's Pat? A woman? A man? Why is Pat in the hospital? Who tramped the message? A child, brother, uncle, friend?

"Everything went well." Jim's voice startles me. I didn't realize he's here.

I'm going to be in the hospital overnight, standard procedure after an axillary dissection. This is my first hospital stay since Joe was born twenty-five years ago. That time I was a new mother and wasn't sick. This time I hurt. It feels as if someone has rammed a dull spear into the left side of my chest.

Later, the night nurse sneaks into my room. The beam of her flashlight bounces across the bed.

"I'm awake," I say. "You can turn on the lights."

"I'm pretty good at working in the dark." She begins to strip the Jackson-Pratt drain that dangles from the left side of my chest. I need to watch her, because when I get home, I'll have to do this myself. Unlike my friend whose husband did it for her, I can't expect Jim to interrupt his work to be my nurse.

She unpins the drain from my hospital gown and, hand over hand, milks the tubing, squeezing the bloody fluid into the clear plastic bulb.

Her identification badge announces her name and rank, "[Something] [Something], PhD, RN."

"Do you have a PhD in nursing?" I ask. Nurses with PhDs usually have administrative or teaching or research jobs. They virtually never work the night shift on the wards.

"No. In chemistry. I received that in my home country, in Syria. In America I became a nurse."

She changes the subject. "It must be awful to have cancer."

"It is."

"Last time I had a mammogram they found calcifications in my breasts." She has just finished taking my blood pressure. "I was so scared I skipped the follow-up appointment."

"You need to have that checked." I shift my weight slightly in the bed. A sharp pain sears my left side. "There are lots of reasons for calcifications in your breasts. It might be something very benign. But, for sure, if it's cancer, you're better off knowing about it."

"Right. I'll take care of that tomorrow."

She finishes stripping the JP. "In the morning I'm going to call for an appointment."

She checks my IV site. She takes my temperature.

As she leaves my room, I remind her, "Be sure you make that call about your mammogram. Tomorrow."

She turns, smiles. "I will. I certainly will."

Who's the patient here, anyway?

During the rest of the night, I drift in and out of wakefulness. There must be a regularity to the rhythm of the SCD—the sequential compression device that is wrapped around each of my legs like children's floaties—but I can't figure it out. The two inflatable air bags are meant to keep clots from forming in my leg veins. It's as if the Mad

Hatter programmed the inflations. Bottom squeeze. Middle squeeze. Bottom release. Top squeeze. Middle release. Top release. The intervals between the cycles seem random. Maybe that's because I wake up at irregular times.

Snip. Snip. Who's trimming their toenails? Snip. Snip. It must be an old man with thick, horny nails. I open my eyes and search the darkened hospital room. No one is here but me. Snip. Snip. I look again. No old man. Nobody. Snip. Snip. Finally it makes sense. The snipping sound is from the machine that inflates the SCD leg wraps.

The next morning, while I'm deciding whether to eat the raspberry jello and vanilla yogurt on my breakfast tray, a friend comes for a visit. She's a physician at the medical center and, it turns out, has had breast cancer. She has brought me several gifts. In one package is a stuffed toy bear with the pink breast cancer logo stitched on the bottom of its paw. In another is a denim cap to wear when my hair falls out.

I unwrap the third package and unroll a yard-long piece of white grosgrain ribbon. "This is the most valuable of all," she says. "You will find that, when you take a shower, you have nowhere to pin the JP drain." She points to the ribbon. "You take off all your clothes, loop the ribbon around your neck, and pin the JP to it." Her smile is broad and knowing.

Later the discharge planning nurse sorts through a pile of papers as she approaches my bed. "Here are the post-op instructions for your mastectomy care," she says.

"But, I didn't have a mastectomy. I had a lumpectomy revision and an axillary node dissection."

"OK." She looks confused and leaves. I never see her again.

The surgery team makes their rounds, but my doctor, Myron, isn't with them. The chief resident is in charge. He summarizes my case for the gaggle of junior residents and medical students who gather around my bed.

"Dr. Gilsdorf," the chief says, "those axillary nodes looked large, a bit larger than I expected."

What's he saying? Is that code for *they looked like they were loaded with cancer?* Why should I have that information? I can do nothing with it until the pathology report is released. Is he speaking to me the doctor or me the patient? I suspect the former. He's young and inexperienced in handling a hybrid physician-patient like me. He'll grow up. He won't be this insensitive forever.

"Ready for a shower? Here you go." A nursing assistant hands me a bar of soap, a towel, and a washrag. "There's a roll of Saran Wrap in the bathroom. Use it to protect your dressings." She leaves the room.

I sit on the edge of the bed and consider my assignment. Other than one staggering trip to the bathroom, I haven't been on my feet at all since my operation. I don't think it's safe yet for me to stumble by myself into the bathroom with only my IV pole for support. Will I be able to stand in the shower long enough to get clean? What if I fall? What if I faint? And, how the hell am I supposed to get the Saran Wrap around my chest? My left arm is useless.

Yesterday I took a shower without effort, without fear. Today a shower has become impossibly difficult and overwhelmingly scary. Slipping my legs back under the bedsheets and laying my head on the pillow, I decide to skip the shower. I'll wash after I get home.

Why do these things happen? If this is the "customer service" provided to faculty physicians—who are more willing to complain than regular patients—what occurs with the others? Or, maybe the nursing staff assume that an infectious diseases pediatrician knows all there is to know about post-op breast cancer care. Well, they are wrong.

※

The next morning, after coming home from the hospital, I'm ready to take a bath but not to stand in the shower. My white grosgrain ribbon rests on the bathroom counter. With my right hand, I pull apart the Velcro that holds my elastic dressing together. As the bandages fall away from my body, I stare at my chest.

"Jim," I scream. "Jim."

My husband races into the bathroom. "What's wrong?" he yells.

"Where's my nipple? It's gone. They weren't supposed to cut off my nipple. Where is it?" My knees wobble and my head spins.

Jim pulls away the rest of the elastic dressing. My nipple is there, but not where it used to be, not where I expected it to be. I stagger to our bed, icy sweat puddling on my forehead, the black drape of an impending swoon fluttering around me.

So this is the "new me," the carved up, displaced, asymmetrical "new me." My sweaty head drenches the pillow. This can't be true. Somehow I must have it all wrong. Soon I'll wake up and this will all be gone.

After the near blackout passes, after I've rested for a while, after I've taken a bath and have reexamined my chest again, I draw a picture of my new anatomy in my journal.

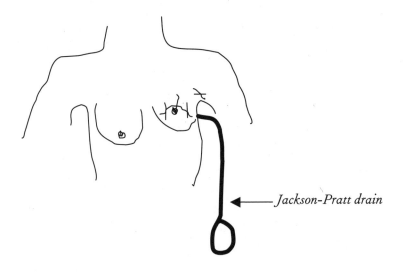

*Jackson-Pratt drain*

Mutilation from an operation ranges from the insignificant, such as a short, faint scar, to the devastating, such as amputation of a limb or deformation of a face. Disfigurement of a breast rests somewhere in between. Its exact position on the mutilation scale varies, dependant on the way the victim views her body, views her life. I can't tell where, ultimately, the "new me" will fall on my personal mutilation scale. At the moment, I give it a high number—a terrible score.

Several days later, Myron calls. "I've got good news and good news. Which do you want to hear first?" he asks.

"You choose."

"The lumpectomy re-excision showed no residual cancer. Also, we harvested fifteen lymph nodes, and none of them are positive."

I page Jim immediately to tell him. If the axillary dissection had revealed more positive nodes, in addition to the single positive one on the sentinel node biopsy, my ultimate prognosis would have been more dismal. This is very good news.

Jim skips into the kitchen after work. "Thanks so much for calling," he says, planting a kiss on my cheek. He settles into his La-Z-Boy and pulls me into his lap. "You know," he says, "I've been haunted by thoughts of spending the rest of my life without you. I imagine bouncing our grandchildren on my knee and you're not there to enjoy them."

His face is solemn; his voice cracks as he speaks. Poor guy. This is tearing him apart.

I love the idea of grandchildren, of Jim building wooden toys for them, of me knitting sweaters and baking brownies for them, of Dan's and Joe's kids—blond and blue-eyed and energetic and curious like their fathers were—giddy with excitement to see us. Both of us. I can't comprehend not being around when Jim is a grandfather.

It's been a week since my axillary dissection and I feel horrible, as if someone is ripping the skin and muscles away from the entire left side of my chest. I can't sleep. I don't leave my easy chair. Nothing interests me, not food or knitting or reading. Not even solitaire.

"Jim, I can't understand why I'm so worthless," I complain.

"My dear, you just had an operation."

"I know, but that was a week ago."

Jim chuckles and lays down the fishing magazine he was reading. "It's like this . . ." he begins.

"Think of Ugh-mug the caveman. Ugh-mug gets injured—say he's mauled by a bear—but he's able to crawl back to his cave. His wife helps him climb onto the pile of deerskins beside the fire and brings him warm, rat-meat soup. She washes off his wounds and smears oily fish heads over the worst of them.

"Does Ugh-mug start plotting, immediately, how to get that bear? No. He hides in the back of his cave and has only one thought—self-preservation. He's not interested in other people, in planning his next hunt, in extracting pleasure or productivity from every hour. Basically he's not interested in anything. He gets very defensive and lashes out at every perceived threat. In short, he's not pleasant to be around.

"That's why you can't concentrate, why you can't read a whole paragraph without losing your place. You can't add a column of numbers correctly; you can't play games; you're no longer socially adept. This is a valuable, albeit primitive, survival response, and it happens even if your injury is a neat and clean surgical wound.

"You see, my sweet, Ugh-mug understands better than you, apparently, that healing requires that he redirect all his energy to mending."

Jim pauses a moment and then adds, "For God's sake, Janet, you've been deeply injured."

After my initial irritation at being upstaged by a caveman, I begin to see the wisdom of Jim's words. Unlike cars and computers, injured bodies have millions of self-repair systems that reconnect severed nerves, realign broken bones, plug oozing holes in blood vessels, knit together tattered tissues, chase away infecting microbes, and apparently keep you from misdirecting your energies. I need to let the system do its work.

※

Injured nerves hurt. A lot. In odd ways. It's been two weeks since my axillary dissection, and I'm in my office on a conference call with a committee of the National Board of Medical Examiners. We're discussing the questions I submitted. The JP drain dangles out of my chest, its bulb pinned to the inside of my new blue velour top. Instead of upper-body underwear, I wear a T-shirt inside out. The seams face away from my skin so their edges won't rub against me.

"We really appreciate your willingness to join us," the committee chairman says over the phone. "How do you feel?"

"Other than the fact that my left armpit is on fire, I feel fine."

This, of course, is a lie. I feel terrible—weak, sore, angry, frustrated. Probably also scared of what lies ahead, but that's hard to admit, even to myself. I don't tell the committee that, besides burning, my armpit feels wet all the time and, yet, the gauze I stuff into my axilla stays dry as a cracker. The slightest stimulation, the twist of my waist or the bend of my left elbow or the friction of clothes against my skin, sends jolts of pain through my arm and chest wall. Worms seem to creep through my healing tissues. A whole region of my left chest and upper arm is numb and feels as puffy as a lip after dental Novocain. It's as if someone has shoved a basketball—a basketball covered with razor blades and ultrahot chili sauce—into my armpit.

So, why am I here, at my desk on this conference call? Why am I not in my bed? Because I'm going to be miserable wherever I am, so I might as well fulfill my responsibilities. Crazy as it may be, I still feel guilty that I'm not actually in Philadelphia with the committee. What *is* my threshold for bailing out of my commitments? I don't know, except that I'm really glad I didn't try a round-trip airplane ride, a lonely hotel room, and two days of meetings feeling like this.

Jim reminds me that this pain and the weird sensations are because my intercostobrachial nerve was "sacrificed"—another bad word for patients to hear—in order to fully explore my axilla. This anatomic explanation, while welcome, does nothing to quell my discomfort.

My lumpectomy incision bothers me less than the axillary dissection incision, but every once in a while an electric buzz shoots through what's left of my breast. My raw, cut nerves must be sending out voltaic signals in search of their lost pieces.

A dream: Jim and I are on vacation, on a cruise. As we prepare to board the ship, we walk the grounds of an old plantation-style manor where we stayed for several nights. We're in a foreign country populated by strange animals. To get a closer look, I lean toward a furry creature the color of caramel. He squirms out of his hole, bites me on the hand, and backs down into his hole again.

His bite leaves a match head–sized pit in the web between my left thumb and index finger. Two days later, the pit has morphed into a two-inch-deep pocket. It doesn't hurt, has no drainage. The wound looks pretty clean, but the animal's saliva seems to be eroding my hand. Jim isn't worried at all about my injury and ignores my suggestion that I consult the ship's doctor.

"What'll he do that we can't do?" Jim asks. But "we" are doing nothing, so I suggest we get off the boat and find a local doctor who might know the animal that bit me. A hometown guy might have an antidote for the flesh-eating enzyme that seems to be dissolving my hand.

Jim and I ask several ship employees how to find a local doctor. They don't know.

I wake up. Helplessness and frustration and dread shadow me all day.

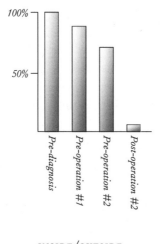

I'm worried that I'll never return to full function at work, that after the surgery and chemo and radiation, not working will become a habit. Or, I worry that I won't give a damn ever again about my research, my teaching, my Pediatric Infectious Diseases division, my patients, because that's the way I feel about them right now. I see the possibilities as all or none—either I work 100 percent of my precancer intensity or zero percent.

In my journal I draw a graph describing how I function at work.

100%

50%

Pre-diagnosis

Pre-operation #1

Pre-operation #2

Post-operation #2

Ten days after my axillary dissection, Myron stares at my scars and asks about the drainage from my JP tube. I hand him my little notebook that shows the steady decrease in the tube's output.

"I think we can pull it out today," he says.

"Good." Then I add, looking down at my asymmetric chest, "I guess my topless dancing days are over. What do you think?"

He chuckles.

# CHAPTER 10

*La morte, la vie*

*This afternoon* I start to read *A Heartbreaking Work of Staggering Genius* by Dave Eggers. It's so beautifully written that I'm breathless as I work my way through the opening pages. Soon I know, as the author and his siblings knew, that the mother is going to die—of cancer— very soon. The dialogue between the author and his mother, who from her bed on the couch deals with nosebleeds and bile and a smart, sassy son, brings me to a stop, over and over. I reread several paragraphs four times, pulling the words from the paper and depositing them in my interior file of lovely prose. In every sentence I see Dan and Joe and me telling jokes, managing life's chores, organizing the household before I leave forever, all the while knotted together by umbilical cords and emotional chains that are stretched to the breaking point.

The pages throb with excruciating details that are at once ordinary and extraordinary, as members of this devastated family, which could easily be the Gilsdorfs, try to comfort each other. Along the way they squabble, resurrect memories, endure disordered bodily functions, move forward in their lives, cope with wrenching endings.

I shut the book and set it on my bedside cabinet. Maybe later. Maybe next month. Maybe next year. All I know is, I can't read it right now.

The phone rings, waking me from a nap. A mature female voice says, "Hello, I'm from Washtenong Memorial Gardens. We're a cemetery and mausoleum . . ." I'm stunned, speechless, can't follow everything she says. Something about a gift certificate.

"Not interested." I'm about to hang up but then add, "This call is very untimely. I've just learned I have breast cancer and now *you* call to have me buried."

She's still apologizing as I return the phone to its cradle.

Maybe this isn't an unbelievably ironic accident. Maybe someone at the hospital is selling names and phone numbers of cancer patients to local cemeteries.

Chin tucks. Shoulder shrugs. Scapula kisses. Ten each. These exercises are part of my physical therapy program after the axillary dissection. If I'm compliant, they will reportedly assure normal functioning of my arm and shoulder. I've set up a little exercise area in our bedroom using the door to the bathroom, the oak coatrack Jim made, and the side chair where Jim used to pile his clothes before the coatrack was built.

To increase the mobility of my left arm, I walk my fingers, spiderlike, up the bathroom door until it hurts, and then a little farther, reaching, reaching, reaching. Then I do ten flexed elbow kisses, ten elbow circles. On the pulley system I rigged up—a length of rope looped over one arm of the coatrack—I pull, teeter-totter fashion, alternately on each end of the rope, ten times. With my arms before me like a shelf I raise my fisted hands over my head, ten times. I do ten arms-only jumping jacks; I can't touch my fingertips together yet—I look like a broken windmill—but I'm making progress.

For arm strength, I do ten push-ups against the bathroom door. Next, I squeeze my clasped hands together and pull them apart ten times, reminiscent of the bosom-building exercises we hopefully, fruitlessly, did at Girl Scout Camp, chanting, "We must, we must, we must enlarge our bust. The bigger the better, the tighter the sweater, the boys depend on us." Finally, gripping a two-pound weight, I swing my left arm backward and then forward to above my head, or at least in that direction, ten times. The weight is a five-pound sack of King Arthur flour, half full.

"You have to do these exercises to prevent a frozen shoulder," the nurse said. I bristled at the words *you have to*, because there is very little that I *have to do*. Rather, I have choices and realize that I will experience the rewards, or consequences, of my choices. I have chosen to do these exercises. I'm not sure what *frozen shoulder* means, but it doesn't sound good. It's a lay term, I guess, that describes reduced range of motion at the shoulder joint, the result of disuse and shortened, inflexible tendons and/or ligaments.

"If you aren't able to do these exercises satisfactorily," the nurse said, "you'll have to go to physical therapy." I definitely don't want to do that.

Another envelope to Joe, bulging with comics and interesting articles, is ready for the mail. As I open the drawer to get a stamp, my gaze cuts across the shelf above and lands on the picture from Dan and Bean's wedding. It was taken by Michael, Dan's former roommate who is now a freelance photographer for a skateboard magazine. The picture captures me at my finest, at one of the happiest moments of my life.

The wedding was last September at the Springton Manor Farm in Chester County, Pennsylvania, a suburb of Philadelphia where Bean's family lives. The night before the ceremony—or before the ceremony was *supposed* to be—Jim and I hosted the rehearsal dinner at the country inn where our friends and relatives were staying. Afterward, we all sat in Grandma Gilsdorf's room drinking wine and joking and laughing and watching, on the TV weather channel, reports of Hurricane Floyd as it crawled up the East Coast.

By morning, it was raining hard and the creeks that ran on either side of our inn had crept over their banks. By noon, the inn was an island. I wrapped my mother-of-the-groom dress in several layers of plastic, preparing to wade through now knee-high water to get to the cars we had moved, earlier, to high ground.

At one o'clock in the afternoon, Bean called to report that the governor had closed all state and county facilities, including the farm and Manor House where the ceremony was to be held.

"The wedding is canceled," she said. Those words reverberated through my head like a death knell. What about all the flowers Bean's sister had arranged? What about the dinner that was probably half-cooked by now? What about Bean's wedding dress? What about the bridesmaids' and flower girl's dresses? What about the cloth napkins we had folded the day before? I paced the narrow hallways of the inn, deeply disturbed that my daughter-in-law's big day was ruined, that the celebration her mother and older sister had planned so carefully was, now, not to be. After every four or five laps I looked out the window at the rain that blew like bullets against the glass. I was helpless at turning off a hurricane.

The water in the yard continued to rise, and the inn's employees left for home before the road was no longer drivable. While eating fruit and muffins from the inn's refrigerators, we played bridge and answered the office phone, telling the callers to check back after the hurricane was over. At 2:30 in the afternoon, Bean called again to tell us the wedding would be the next day, that the Manor House, the gardens, the caterer, the minister, the limousine, and the DJ would all be available.

The following afternoon, the water had receded, the sun shone, and the wedding went on. The day was almost biblical, reminiscent of the moment Noah emerged from the ark.

Michael snapped this photo, the one that sits on the shelf above the stamp drawer, during the marriage ceremony. It's a black and white print, a dramatic close-up of Jim and me. A dewy gardenia is pinned to my jacket. My laughing face, in profile, looks at Jim, who is square with the camera, his gaze off to the side, toward me. A breeze, the last of the wind that blew away Hurricane Floyd, fluffs my hair.

I cradle the photo in my hands. In this picture, I'm beautiful, vibrant, loving, and loved. "Jim," I say, "if I go away, I want you to remember me like this."

I write in my journal:

*Everything takes longer. It's like driving with the emergency brake on.*

"When the Visa bill comes this month," I say to my husband, "sit down before you open it."

"Uh-oh. What did you buy?"

"More clothes."

My cancer wardrobe is expanding. I've discovered that I like my comfy pants and don't look as horrible as I thought in them. This morning I ordered four pairs of slacks: navy linen, ivory linen, dominoes print, and bluefish silkscreen. I also ordered a denim V-necked shirt—the slash of the V modest rather than plunging—with fabric knots instead of buttons and two linen shirt jackets, one ebony and the other barn red.

I suppose there's a psychological explanation for this buying spree. It probably has to do with pretty cover-ups and a mangled body, with shabby self-esteem and an uncertain future. The pictures in the catalogs show slender, active women who seem to live exciting, fun lives. In addition, the models have two intact breasts and, apparently, not a care in the world. Perhaps I'm more vulnerable now to marketing schemes that prey on people's subterranean needs. I want to be the women in the pictures. Maybe if I *look* like them, I can *be* them. Whatever the reason, the hours I spend planning my wardrobe have been very therapeutic. Their feel-good effect is more enduring than two Tylenols.

Yesterday I wore a bra for the first time since my axillary dissection, a testament to my arm's ability to fasten the hooks. It was short-lived. The lateral end of the underwire on the left side dug into my skin. Even wads of Kleenex stuffed between me and the wire didn't help. This afternoon, when Jim and I go to the birdseed store, I'll stop at the sports shop and get a soft jogging bra.

A dream: I'm out of town at a scientific meeting and trying to connect with a car-pool group to go home. The details are fuzzy: what time will we leave? where will we leave from? are we leaving Friday evening or Saturday morning? I stop at the meeting's headquarters to try to get the departure information. The people manning the booth are old high school friends of mine, now grown up. Even though a few of them are in the car pool, they ignore me. They act as if I'm a pesky homeless person begging for money.

I return to my hotel, accompanied by a guy I had a crush on in high school. This fellow, in reality, paid little attention to me back then and, again in reality, is now a family physician somewhere. As we walk in the dream, I gesture toward a tree growing out of a grate in the sidewalk. My outstretched arm is dotted with circular red spots—many of them—as if I've been strafed with bird shot.

I rub the spots and say, "Looks like erythema multiforme."

My friend glances at the spots and says, "Yup. You must have a gammopathy (abnormal proteins in the blood) or something." We continue toward the hotel, both aware of the unspoken—that the spots are an immune reaction from my cancer, that they may or may not signify something bad.

Someone is being buried in the Dixboro Village cemetery. A hearse waits in the lane beside the fence, and cars line both sides of Plymouth Road. The cemetery, a quarter mile from our house, is small and filled with aged tombstones. This burial must be in the last empty grave in the lot.

Although I drive this stretch several times a day—past the old Dixboro School, past the Dixboro Store, past the maple trees that lined the road back when it was a winding gravel path—I have paid little attention to the cemetery. Today, I see it as I never have before. The official name is Oak Grove Cemetery, and, indeed, it is nestled beside Fleming Creek in a shady woodlet of old pine and oak trees.

I think about the birds. From inside my car, I can't see or hear them, but I know they're here. The same birds that come to our feeders—the goldfinches, cardinals, house finches, jays—undoubtedly fly through the treetops from our yard to this cemetery. Probably even Blackie—the cardinal with a featherless, ebony head—spends time here. Except for the traffic on Plymouth Road, this would be a lovely place to rest forever.

If I die of my cancer, would I be buried here? Jim and I have never talked about our own funerals. When it comes to something as permanent as burial, this may not be the right place. To me, Michigan doesn't exactly seem like home but rather like an eighteen-year stopover. Where *would* I be buried? North Dakota, where I grew up? Minnesota, where I was born and where we lived for three years before moving to Michigan? California, where we lived twenty-five years ago but where I still have a license to practice medicine? I guess Jim and I are nomads, without roots. Where are nomads buried? Some on Boot Hill, some at sea, some in any old hole in the ground.

Except for earlier today when I drove past the funeral, I don't think much about dying. Denial of the possible ultimate outcome of my cancer is adaptive and serves me well. Jim, on the other hand, thinks about my dying a lot.

"You're awfully quiet tonight," I say.

Jim, grasping a glass of bourbon, slumps in his La-Z-Boy. "Yeah."

"Why?"

"You don't want to know."

"Of course I want to know. If you don't tell me, I'll imagine the worst. Are you about to file for divorce?"

"No." He takes a sip of his drink. He takes a deep breath. He takes another sip. "One of my breast cancer patients came in today with a backache." He takes yet another sip of the bourbon. "Her spine films showed a bone met."

"Oh," I say quietly. "Jim, it's OK to tell me these things. I know the possibilities, know they happen to other women and might happen to me. Please don't quit talking to me."

Jim had several vacation trips planned for this summer. One by one, he has canceled the fishing excursion to the Bahamas and the trip to Michigan's Upper Peninsula and has rescheduled the bamboo fly rod–building workshop. His brother John calls and suggests they postpone the Gilsdorf family horseback, fly-fishing trip to Montana.

"We can do it next year, Jim," John says.

"Absolutely not," I say. "That trip will not be postponed because of me. It's been planned for a year, and eight people have their reservations all made. Besides, Jim, you need brother therapy *really* bad."

A social work intern from the Cancer Center calls to inform me of their support services. Her name is Sarah, a sweet, well-meaning, kind-person name. She describes "Reach for Recovery," a one-on-one program matching an experienced "breast cancer survivor"—one who has emerged from the other side—with "a woman currently on treatment"—one still dog-paddling through the mire. She also describes several support group options.

I'm not interested. It's the elitist in me. I would probably feel different about a support group if Sarah could guarantee that the members would be university faculty women with cancer. I fear I would have little in common with most women in a regular group because I come from a different perspective. The other women might, understandably, be terrified about things I'm not scared of, such as IVs and the medical equipment and the system in general. For them, the unknowns that surround each aspect of their treatment are vast. I, on the other hand, am familiar with the biology of cancer as well as with surgical routines and chemotherapy and the rudiments of radiation; I provide medical care, after all, to children with cancer who get frequent and weird and serious infections.

Other women may cling to promises of "miracle drugs," to the superiority of "the best cancer doctor." I know there are no such things. Like other women, I need my physicians to be caring and knowledgeable and to treat me as an individual rather than "that breast cancer in room 7." But women sometimes up the ante and become unrealistically dependent on their physicians. Sometimes they need their doctors to be omnipotent. We physicians, of course, foster some of the medical omnipotency mystique, because the correct amount is, in truth, part of the therapeutic contract. I, however, understand the boundaries of patient-doctor relationships, know what doctors can do for me—give sound medical advice—and what they cannot do—be my mother, my best friend, my favorite uncle. My doctors cannot erase every unhappiness that clouds my life.

I'm sure my presence in a support group would alter the group interactions. Knowing me, I would end up taking care of the other group members. I might even outlead the group leader.

Sarah goes on to describe the "Look Good, Feel Better" program, a two-hour class to teach women to be beautiful during chemotherapy: how to cope with the hair thing, what to do about missing eyebrows and eyelashes, how to use makeup to cover raccoon eyes and God knows whatever else will be wrong with my skin.

While the other support groups don't interest me at all, this one does. A little.

I call my friend Trudy, a pediatric infectious diseases physician in Georgia. She concurs that support groups aren't for everyone.

"Maybe, though, if you joined," she says, "you could come to see your differences, the ones between you and the group, as background shadows, and the spotlight could shine on your common concerns." She agrees that I would likely take care of the other members of the group but thinks that might be good for me. She's talking about a kind of transference in which my needs are satisfied by giving to others what I need most. That doesn't sound healthy or in my best interest.

I decide to attend the "Look Good, Feel Better" class as a trial balloon for a support group. We gather at the Cancer Center with a social worker, a cosmetologist who volunteers her time, and a stack of makeup boxes donated by cosmetics companies. As an introduction, they show a video narrated by an upbeat, gorgeous, professional woman who is elegantly dressed, beautifully coifed, and made up like a model. She introduces herself as a cancer patient and explains the goals of the program. An oncologist—male—discusses the importance of self-esteem in coping with cancer and cancer treatments. At the end of the video, the beautiful narrator lifts off her beautiful hair to reveal a bald chemo head.

Four other patients sit at the table with me. I size them up. All appear to be between thirty-five and fifty-five years old.

Julia is a carefully dressed, aloof woman who recently had her first chemotherapy treatment and is beginning to lose her lovely, flowing-like-a-river-of-gold hair. She appears to be a professional woman and seems mad at the world.

Michelle is more funky, more flexible, than Julia. She seems to be the Common Woman: fun and down-to-earth.

Laurie's hair is a tangerine tangle, and her makeup is garish. She appears streetwise and definitely has an attitude.

Trish is on her third round of chemo and is completely bald. She is neither sophisticated nor highly educated but is honest and deeply sincere. She will surely die of her cancer but, although she's clawing up a steep cliff, to her credit she's still trying.

The social worker asks for someone to volunteer to be made up. With our hands in our laps, we avoid her stare. Finally, I raise my arm—the right one, the one that can be raised—and say, "Sure, you can demonstrate on me."

Julia and Laurie came to class heavily made up, so they just sit and watch. Michelle and Trish take their cues from the cosmetologist, who applies moisturizer, foundation, rouge, mascara, eyeliner, and lipstick to me. Then they gamely practice on themselves.

Could I be in a true support group with them? Maybe with Julia, as she is obviously well educated, but she's too sullen, too private. Could a support group be like my book group? I doubt it. My book group emerged from established friendships and is built upon our love of reading and discussing fiction rather than upon a random disaster that has struck us all. In the support group, there would be no selection for age, educational level, interests, values, or worldviews. It would be like taking the next seven people in line at the post office and, with no identifiable affinities, forcing them to be friends. I don't think cancer alone is the right affinity for me to join a group.

*La morte, la vie*

Mike, a veterinarian turned radiologist, and Jim were good friends—fellow physicians who bragged about being the most "sartorially challenged" doctors in their hospital. Between OR cases, Jim would read Mike's *Detroit Free Press* by the light of the view boxes while Mike read x-ray films. Occasionally they would share lunch and fishing tales with another of their buddies, the janitor.

Now Mike is dead. He opted for a stent to fix his stenotic coronary artery and, forty-eight hours later, ended up with a dissecting aneurysm. After two hellish weeks on life support, Mike died at the age of fifty-eight.

If there is such a thing as a lovely day for a funeral, this is it. The sun warms the clouds as they bob like cotton balls in the clear blue sky. This is the first funeral I have attended with Jim in thirty years of marriage, not counting the visitation for a colleague's teenage daughter who worked in my lab one summer and then took her own life.

Mike's wife, flanked by their two young sons, greets us at the chapel door. She grasps my hands and thanks me warmly for coming. In spite of the enormity of her loss, she seems to be comforting me in my illness. The irony is dazzling . . . I have cancer, Mike is dead. Hundreds of people jam the sanctuary. Jim and I take the last two seats.

The ceremony is both beautiful and heart wrenching. His friends and medical colleagues speak of Mike the doctor, the husband, the father; of Mike the hunter, sailor, biker, tinkerer, woodworker, soccer coach. Someone reads an essay written by one of Mike's sons—an English class assignment. Someone else reads a passage from the book of Psalms, then one from Ecclesiastes.

"For every thing there is a season . . ." It's been many years, going back to my Lutheran catechism days, since I've heard these familiar passages. Their words, poetic and simple, ring with the rhythms of life. Their beauty, and the wisdom of the one who wrote them, humbles me. I clutch Jim's hand.

The line to the casket for a last good-bye to Mike is slow moving. As we approach, I focus on the white, pleated satin that lines the coffin.

Shiny. Smooth. Soft. Mike's eternal bunk. This berth doesn't seem right for Mike. He ought to be hunkered down in the bottom of an oar boat, a tackle box at his feet, a fishing rod in one hand, a beer in the other. What would it be like to lie on that satin? What would it be like to have the lid of the casket close, to be entombed in darkness, forever, on that glossy, white, pleated bed?

The man in the coffin isn't Mike; the lifeless fellow in the box has no devious twinkle in his eye, no sarcastic grin, no wild-haired character. The Mike we knew laughed all the time, was cynical as hell, was brilliant, was kind.

At home after the funeral and the interment, Jim and I sit in silence. We can't share our thoughts, for they are too overwhelming to be cast in words. Surreal as Mike's death seems, its reality is absolute, as if our tent has collapsed and we are suffocating, as if our canoe has sunk and we are drowning.

Hopefully a metastasis won't do me in, but the pain in my left axilla might. I can't sleep; it aches, it stings, it feels as if a hound has chomped on my armpit and is ripping out a hunk of flesh. Even though I detest taking medicine, I called in a prescription for Neurontin and have taken it for about a week. The pain—the burning, the ripping—is still there, though, and the drug makes me fuzzy, as if I'm living in a watercolor rather than in a finely detailed still life. I try a Clonidine patch, and that also does nothing for the pain.

I didn't expect neuraesthesias (abnormal sensations) of this degree, wasn't warned about them. This particular complication wasn't mentioned when I signed the op permit for the axillary dissection. Then, the resident read off the list of adverse effects: pain, blood loss, wing scapula (if they inadvertently cut the long thoracic nerve), numb upper arm (if they cut the intercostobrachial nerve), and death. Nothing about armpit being on fire for weeks on end.

Thoughts of dying, written in my journal:

*God commissions St. Peter to develop a five-year plan. A month later, St. Peter presents it to God. God flips through the pages and notes my name.*

*"Oh, for Christ's sake," God exclaims. "I have enough trouble. I don't need that Gilsdorf woman here in Heaven stirring up more. Leave her in Ann Arbor."*

# CHAPTER 11

*Kill My Cancer but Don't Kill Me*

*The placard above the registration window* in the infusion suite reads "CHECK IN HERE," and a thick maroon arrow points to a clipboard on the shelf below. As instructed, I write my name, the time of my appointment, and the time of my arrival on the sign-in sheet. The last column is labeled "Port or Broviac?" I write "NO."

Port or Broviac . . . I haven't given a thought to intravenous access for the chemotherapy drugs. I stare at the back of my right hand, at the web of blood-filled hoses that jut from my skin like an elm branch in bas-relief. If the nurse can't get an IV started in one of those, she needs to go back to nursing school.

Jim and I find seats in the crowded waiting room. I pull my knitting from my bag and settle it in my lap. The wool is variegated in shades of olive green, navy blue, and deep purple. I'm on a purl row, and every stitch is different in color from the last. Jim pages through a *Sports Afield* magazine.

As I switch from the purl row to a knit row, I look up from my needles. The man beside me is the color of a dull nickel and the one across the aisle the color of a muddy egg yolk. No one looks healthy. The patients are ill, and their family members are sad.

Soon I'll be one of them, a chemotherapy recipient. The people in this waiting room disturb me. Their strained faces speak of faded hope and ongoing anguish, of uncertainty, of resignation, of despair. I knit faster, my eyes riveted to the yarn that twists through my fingers, loops over the needles, and settles into yet another stitch in the growing textile.

Earlier this morning I had an appointment with my oncologist. He reviewed the plan for my chemotherapy—Adriamycin and Cytoxan for four cycles and then Taxol for four more cycles.

"Do you suffer from motion sickness when you travel?" he asked as he wrote the dosages on the order sheet.

"Yes."

"Did you have morning sickness with your pregnancies?"

"Yes."

"Well, Janet," he said slowly, "you may have a bit more trouble with nausea from the drugs."

More trouble? More trouble than what? More than is safe? Than is bearable? More than 95 percent of cancer patients have?

"Be sure you drink enough water," he said.

"Eat only a light lunch today" were his final words.

The medical literature on breast cancer is massive. The number of published papers that describe the biology, epidemiology, risks, diagnosis, treatment, and prevention of this disease is daunting, and the background knowledge required to understand them is legendary. After my cancer was diagnosed, I downloaded several reviews of breast cancer from the university's online library. From my reading I gained a general sense of what I'm about to go through and have learned the following:

- Chemotherapy improves survival.
- Using several chemotherapy drugs is better than using only one. These drugs work in different ways; they poison different metabolic pathways in my cells. It's like attacking the weeds in the garden with a broad-leaf herbicide as well as a grass killer.
- Twelve months of chemo is no better than six months of the same drugs.
- Anthracycline-containing drugs—such as Adriamycin, the A in the A-C combination—may give a slight survival advantage over other combinations, but it's more toxic.

Adriamycin is more likely to cause hair loss, a consideration that pales in the face of survival versus nonsurvival. Also, this drug is toxic to the heart, which clearly may handicap people, permanently, or may kill them.
- Tamoxifen improves survival in women with ER/PR positive cancers, and five years of it does so better than merely one year.

The data I read represent an overview. They predict what may happen among, say, one hundred women who have breast cancer. They do not, however, predict what *will* happen to *each* woman, what *will* happen to *me*.

In recognition of this uncertainty, the standard is to treat breast cancer aggressively, to offer chemotherapy to any patient who has greater than a 10 percent likelihood of dying from her breast cancer in the next ten years. Under these guidelines, a small number of women who might benefit from treatment won't get it. On the other hand, a larger number of women who wouldn't die from their cancer within ten years will be treated and, thus, may be exposed to the toxicity while receiving only limited benefit. The problem is that among one hundred women with breast cancer sitting in a cancer center waiting room—young, old, black, white, yellow, brown, skinny, fat, rich, poor—no one can tell for sure which ones are likely to profit from chemotherapy.

As far as I can tell from my situation with a positive axillary node and a two-centimeter tumor, the chemotherapy may improve my chance of survival by 6 to 12 percent. That's a low number, considering the toxicity of the drugs. Yet, staying alive absolutely trumps dying. Many other, unknowable factors weigh into the equation of my outcome, such as the subtle biologic characteristics of my cancer that can't be measured, so the actual benefit to me of chemotherapy remains an educated guess, at best.

What do I do? Accept the possible benefit, absolute magnitude unknown, of chemotherapy? That means also accepting the side effects of the drugs, which vary from person to person but, eerily, are more certain, or at least more measurable, than the benefits.

I'm sitting here in the infusion center because I have opted for what my oncologist has suggested. I'm about to receive the chemo.

"JANET GILSDORF." My name rings through the waiting room. I gather my knitting and walk toward the voice.

"I'm Alice and I'll be your nurse during your chemotherapy treatment." The middle-aged woman wearing high-water pants and an often-washed blouse smiles warmly. "Please come with me."

Jim and I follow her into the infusion area, to an empty olive-colored leatherette Strato-Lounger. "Have a seat," Alice says.

On either side of me, the row of green Strato-Loungers arcs beneath a bank of curved windows. Most of the chairs are occupied. The people who fill them are the weary, the wasted, the hairless, the old, the cancerous. I tilt my Strato-Lounger back, and Jim sits in the chair near my feet.

Alice brings the IV equipment, pulls up a stool, ties a tourniquet around my right arm, and easily inserts a needle into my vein. As she works, I notice that her fingers are deft, her hands scaly. Too much soap? Too much chemo?

"I need a dosage check," Alice yells toward the nurses' station. One of her colleagues scurries over to confirm that both the pharmacy and Alice have prepared the medicine as my oncologist ordered. This is a relatively new safety measure at our hospital, instituted after an adverse event surrounding chemo administration. In some ways, the fact that an accident prevention protocol is in place is reassuring. On the other hand, it's a reminder that medical mistakes happen at the best of places.

My chemo is ready to go. Alice turns the valve on my IV, and Adriamycin, bright red and shimmering like rubies in the clear plastic tubing, begins to flow into my body. Drip. Drip. The rhythm of fate. Drip. Drip.

It's noisy in the infusion room. A television hangs from the ceiling between alternate Strato-Loungers. I don't watch TV—ever—so I have no interest in this one. Most of the sets are turned on. The employees are noisy, too. They tell jokes, laugh, put on an upbeat façade. Is this effort to deal with terminally ill patients sincere, or is it just an act? Is it their awkward way of protecting themselves from unending disease? Whatever the reason, it doesn't feel real or appropriate to me. The staff members seem like a troupe of aerialists, lion tamers, acrobats, jugglers, and snake charmers that took a wrong turn and, instead of the circus tent, ended up in the infusion room.

There are lots of hugs. Hugs between nurses and patients for starting chemo, for finishing chemo, for just being there. Nurses hug each other. I don't get a hug for starting chemo; I think my body language tells them to tone it down with me. The hilarity of the staff is in marked contrast to the moods of the patients—glum, forlorn, fed up.

Two hours later, the bag of Adriamycin hooked to my IV is almost empty. The drug is now circulating inside me, percolating through every capillary bed, soaking every cell. The deed is done. The first dose is complete. My hair will fall out. I've got three to four weeks before the unthinkable happens.

Something lands in my left eye. Probably an eyelash or a piece of mascara. Blinking doesn't remove it. Neither does rubbing. Alice puts her arms around me and gives me a hug. Apparently she thinks I'm wiping away tears. I guess I am, but they are tears from an irritated cornea, not tears from crying.

Alice hooks up the bag of my second drug, Cytoxan. "I need a dosage check," she yells again.

The infusion ends without incident. Driving home, Jim says, "I'm starved." It's two o'clock in the afternoon and we have had no lunch.

I feel pretty good. In fact, I'm buzzed from the steroids I took yesterday and again just before the infusion this morning. Jim pulls into a Middle Eastern diner.

He orders a plateful of food, and, at first, I order only a cup of tea. But the garlic and chickpeas and cumin and sesame seeds smell so good. And I feel fine. "Eat light," my oncologist had said. So I order a small piece of spinach pie.

Adriamycin (whose real name is doxorubicin), the red liquid that dripped into my vein and now makes my urine pink, is among the anthracycline family of anticancer drugs. Anthracycline. Sounds like coal, looks like cranberry juice. It works as a topoisomerase inhibitor; these words make me think of a fuchia-headed, floppy-footed Bozo the Clown. Adriamycin shuts down the ability of my DNA to unspool and, thus, to reproduce. In short, it's birth control for cancer cells.

Like the seasons, cells cycle: M phase (mitosis/dividing), G1 phase (growth), S phase (DNA synthesis), and G2 phase (growth again). Round and round and round, as regular as the turning of the earth. Adriamycin stops the cycle of the cells in the M or S phase.

The bad news is that Adriamycin doesn't affect only cancer cells but attacks the DNA replication machinery in *all* my cells. Those that take the biggest hit are the ones that divide rapidly, cancer cells as well as blood cells, intestinal tract cells, and hair follicles. That explains the side effects: hair loss; mouth sores, nausea, and vomiting; decreased red blood cells (which carry oxygen to my tissues), white blood cells (which fight infection), and platelets (which help my blood clot and keep me from bleeding all over the place). It causes skin ulcers if the IV leaks out of my vein. And it may damage my heart. That's what happened to a woman who was homecoming queen two classes behind me at Fargo High School; she died, as an adult, of heart failure from Adriamycin treatment of her cancer.

Cytoxan (whose real name is cyclophosphamide) is an alkylating agent. Sounds chemical, sounds harsh. Similar to bubble gum fallen into a pile of string, Cytoxan tangles the strands of my DNA so it no longer unspools. The DNA, then, can't reproduce itself, and the cells die. Again, this affects all my DNA, in all my cells. The side effects are similar to those of Adriamycin: hair loss, decreased blood cells, nausea, vomiting, loss of appetite. In addition, this drug causes bladder irritation and a metallic taste in the mouth. Hair loss is the first item on the complications lists because, like the first ingredient on a soup can label, *it is major*, particularly to women.

An hour after we get home, I begin to feel queasy. "Think I'll lie down," I say to Jim and head for bed, our orange mixing bowl tucked under my arm. Shortly, the spinach pie and everything else in my stomach come up. As I stare at the green flakes swirling among the mucus in the orange bowl, I decide the spinach pie wasn't such a great idea after all.

I toss and turn all night, my left arm aching, my stomach churning, my head throbbing. At dawn, the early morning birds start to chirp. I drift in and out of sleep, vaguely aware that Jim gets up. He plants a kiss on my cheek and leaves to make hospital rounds.

About nine o'clock in the morning, the phone rings. It's my oncologist, checking up on me.

"How're you doing?"

"I'm fine," I say, wishing it were really true. "I had a little vomiting but seem to be OK now."

"Be sure you drink enough fluids."

After several hours—or is it several days, weeks, years, for I can't tell; time has no meaningful dimensions now—Jim returns home and empties the mixing bowl again. "Here, honey, drink some water." He holds a glass to my lips. I choke down a couple swallows.

By the next morning, I've been in my nightgown for thirty-six hours and have crawled out of bed four times to go the eight steps to the toilet. In my journal, barely able to hold a pen, I write:

*Too sick. Too sick. Too sick.*

Now it's forty-eight hours since my infusion, and I'm miserable. Listless as a rag. Head pounding. Too weak to sit up. Too hot. Too cold. Fingers tingle. Toes tingle. Left arm sore as hell. I can't get comfortable no matter what I try and can barely get a few sips of water down. Still in my nightgown, I haven't brushed my teeth or taken a shower for two days.

"Honey," Jim says, his face gray, "I think we should take you to the emergency room." He sounds as miserable as I feel.

"Why?"

"Because you look like shit."

"No." I rearrange my pillow. "I'm not bleeding anywhere. I'm still breathing. My heart's still ticking. I've been able to drink a little and am still urinating. Let me sleep."

Instead of sleeping, though, I weave in and out of strange states of dreaming. Rather than illusory scenes or plots, my mind is cluttered with repetitive thought fragments.

A pilot light at the end of a tunnel. A pilot light at the end of a tunnel.

The deck is full. The deck is full. The deck is full.

The water is verdant. The water is verdant. The water is verdant.

The water is warm. The water is warm.

Chosen. Chosen. Chosen. Chosen.

It's Monday morning—my chemo infusion was Friday—and Jim has gone to work. I stumble to the bathroom and realize that I'm feeling a little better. I haven't vomited for twelve hours and, even though I'm standing up, I don't feel like I'm going to faint.

It's time for a bath.

The water in the tub, silky from the fragrant salts my daughter-in-law sent me, feels like gossamer against my tingling skin. The steamy air smells of jasmine. My precancer routine was to scramble out of bed, take an eight-minute shower with hair wash and rinse, get dressed, put on eye makeup, dash out the door, and drive like a rabid bat to my office at the university. Today I'm floating in the bathtub, following my friend Margaret's recommendation on how to be sick: "Lay low 'til you feel better, then get up."

After my bath, I take a nap.

After the nap, I iron away the creases from three pairs of new pants and rearrange the sheets in the upstairs linen closet. Then I take another nap.

I try a game of solitaire. Somehow I have strung five red cards together in a run. They're supposed to alternate black and red. I stare at the playing cards arrayed before me. I can't figure out what I did, can't remember how to play this game. Just a week ago I won every fourth hand.

Time is sooooooooo slow. When will Jim come home? I don't want the radio on. We never watch television. I don't want any noise.

The daffodils beside the pond in the backyard are beginning to bloom; their sunny faces waver in the breeze. For the past three hours, two male mallards have sat, shoulder to shoulder, at the edge of the water. No female is in sight. Maybe we have a pair of gay ducks. That's OK, they can stay here. There's room in our yard for animals of any persuasion.

A morbidly obese squirrel, fat from raiding the bird feeder, has wedged himself, upright, into the crotch of the beech tree outside the family room window. Pok, pok, pok, pok. He gnaws on an acorn, his front paws around the nut as if in prayer. His little testicles hang like fruit between his thighs. If the window weren't between us, I could reach out and tickle his tummy.

The words of this month's *Atlantic* magazine swim across the page. I can't follow their meaning, can't hold more than two or three of them in my head at one time. Looking at pictures in catalogs still works, though. Sort of.

Finally, Jim comes home.

"Want something to eat?" His hand grasps the open refrigerator door. He stoops and explores its contents.

"God, no."

He cuts a piece of cheese and then eats a plateful of taco chips, dunking each one into a jar of salsa.

He looks forlornly at me in my easy chair. "Janet, we've been married nearly thirty years and I've never seen you just sitting."

That's right. I'm just sitting. Not knitting, not reading, not talking, not playing solitaire. Just sitting.

❧

Claire calls this morning. She asks about my chemo, so I explain that I received the first of four cycles of Adriamycin and Cytoxan and then I will get a four-cycle course of Taxol as well.

"What does Taxol do to you?" she asks.

"Myalgia, arthralgia, peripheral neuropathy, neutropenia, alopecia . . ." I recite the litany of side effects. "But, I'll already have alopecia from the Adriamycin."

She has misheard me and thinks I said the alopecia has arrived.

"Your hair hasn't fallen out already, has it?" She sounds alarmed.

"Not yet," I say, "but I'm ready."

*Kill My Cancer but Don't Kill Me*

"No, you're not."

Her sharp words hit the bull's-eye. I may have the straw hats and silk flowers, but that's different from being ready. "You're right," I admit.

A heron sits high on a tree behind the pond. At first I thought his blue-gray back was a burl on the tree limb. Slowly, he rises to his feet, unfolds his wings, floats down to the side of the pond, and marches on stick-thin legs over the grass to behind the pine tree. The sun, angled from the west, shines off his slate-colored feathers while huge, wet snowflakes flutter out of the sky. A hint of spring, a memory of winter.

I'm ready for something to eat. A scrambled egg might be good: protein, bland, simple to make, small amount. I melt a teaspoon of butter in my smallest skillet; sauté a chopped scallion, including the green part for color; and stir in an egg. It smells luscious, reminds me of breakfast at my Grandma Reed's house when I was a little girl.

The scent follows my fork to my mouth, but once inside, its buttery odor changes to a vile taste, and I can barely swallow the first bite. It's like eating grass clippings soaked in motor oil. The second bite is no better. The rest of the egg goes down the disposal.

The oily grass taste won't go away. I brush my teeth three times, but it still lingers.

Several days ago, Emmy brought a kettle of homemade chicken soup. Even though it, as does everything else, tastes metallic, it's a meal from Heaven. I've discovered that lemonade helps cut through the brassy taste. I expect I'll drink an ocean of it before this is over. Today I try a piece of the cornbread Emmy brought. It's too coarse. Won't go down. Sticks in my gullet.

Now that the chicken soup is gone, I decide to boil a potato. Cradling it in my hands, I slip into reverie, back to our Indian reservation days. A wood-sided, flatbed truck rumbled down Highway 51 from Idaho into town and stopped in front of our house. A crusty farmer, his leather face ridged from the sun and his fingers coated with soil, rang the doorbell.

"D'ya need any spuds?" he asked.

"Sure," I answered.

Moments later he hauled a one-hundred-pound gunny sack stuffed with Idaho russet potatoes, each the size of a hiking boot, up the driveway.

"Want 'em in the garage?" he called. The dry, high mountain desert breeze, fresh off the chokecherry bushes that grew in the lava beds on the hillside, ruffled the legs of his overalls as he walked up the driveway.

"Thanks," I said. Those were such simple, healthy times.

My potato, only three inches long, is finished cooking. I slice it open, rub butter over the flaky, cut surface, and sprinkle chopped parsley on top. It's a feast for a king. Still, it tastes like oily grass with an overtone of aluminum.

I need a few things from the grocery store, so I take my first field trip out of the house since my chemo infusion five days ago. Busch's supermarket is only a mile down the road, but I'm very uncertain driving my car. I pause at every intersection to be sure someone isn't about to ram into my side; I stop at every green light to be sure it's really green.

I fill the cart: eggs and a sack of potatoes; milk, dry cereal, and ice cream for Jim; a chicken and the makings for more homemade soup; a bag of fresh lemons. By the time I reach the checkout lane, my knees are wobbly.

At home, I set the grocery bags on the kitchen counter and ache for bed. If I lie down now, however, the ice cream will melt all over the other food. So, as they say in physical therapy, I push, push, push until it hurts and then push a little more, and soon all the groceries are put away. Then I take a nap.

My research laboratory meeting is this morning, as it has been every Thursday for at least ten years. I want to go very much but don't dare drive that far. I want to hear what everyone is doing—how Melinda's subtraction hybridization experiments are going, whether Rich has isolated the component of *H. influenzae* that turns on inflammatory mediators, whether Jingping's dot blots are working this week. I want to do what I usually do with them on Thursday mornings—hear the results of the week's experiments and decide how to iron out the wrinkles. My good buddy Carl is standing in for me. Maybe next week I'll be able to go.

Since I still can't read, I study catalogs and discover that the ribbed Italian water glasses I have always admired in the Metropolitan Museum of Art are on sale. I call to place an order. An electronic voice answers and puts me on hold. I'm very impatient with waiting and begin chopping onions and carrots for the chicken soup. When the catalog representative finally answers to take my order, I slam the chef's knife against the chopping block so she can hear that I'm busy. It's a bit of theater, but being busy makes me feel good. For about four minutes, I'm multitasking—chopping vegetables, drinking lemonade, and placing a catalog order. Almost like normal. I want the museum employee, the lady with the heavy Boston accent whom I imagine to be the assistant curator, to know that the woman on the phone from Michigan is busy.

# Chapter 12

## *Rapunzel, Rapunzel...*

*Day after day, in the morning* when I brush my teeth and again at bedtime, I stare with disbelief into the bathroom mirror. The person I've always known as me stares back. That reflected lady is going to change. She's going to be bald.

I rake my fingers through my hair. It glides like silk threads against my skin, and the bathroom light sparkles off each strand; my hair is a crazy quilt of yellowy-brown colors: cashew, dun, maple sugar, weak tea. I turn to the left, turn to the right, then face forward. Again, I check the profile, the oblique right, the oblique left. What will it be like without hair?

When I was in seventh grade, Miss Sanford, the old-maid guidance counselor, told us to write a paragraph entitled "What's Good about Me." I was stumped. Couldn't think of a single thing. I, forever the Dora Do-Right student, was caught in a trap—I had an assignment but nothing to write about. Everything about me seemed average; nothing seemed good. Finally I remembered that someone had once said I had nice hair. So I wrote, *Some people say I have nice hair. When I was little, it was platinum* [my mother's word for the color] *and fell in soft ringlets down my back. Now it is darker blond and not curly at all.* My one good feature. Soon it will be gone.

I stare into the mirror, at the honey-colored mane that has framed my face for over fifty years. What will I look like without it? Contemplating the image before me, I try to erase the left-flopping cowlick and the tufts at the sides that I sometimes tuck behind my ears. The visual subtraction doesn't work; I can't conjure up a picture of the lady in the mirror without hair.

I shut my eyes, obliterate the view of the looking glass, block out the world. It's unspeakably horrid. My heart races. I need to run. Bald. Me, bald. The thought is a deep-throated, animalistic howl, like a frantic, screaming plea in the dead of the night. It's the menacing, grotesque, impossible-to-embrace inevitability that faces us all. It's my fate; I will really die. I will really lose my hair. It will really, really, can't-escape-by-any-possible-means happen.

I keep busy, planting pansies in garden pots on the deck; filling the bird feeders; going to work when I feel up to it; working from home on the computer when I don't dare drive. These things fill the time, focus my attention on the here and now, dispatch the darkest thoughts. But the surreal, icy fact remains that my hair will fall out, and soon.

Jim's brother Walt and his wife, Barb, are driving to Michigan from Syracuse, New York, for a visit. Their trip was in limbo for several days because of Barb's sore back, but now they are on their way. I'm VERY excited about having company.

During my rest times, I lie on my bed and prepare for visitors. I plan what I'll cook, how I'll haul my mother's china up from the basement for one meal, will use my wedding china for another. I consider removing every weed in the garden, washing the windows, baking bread, buying new sheets for the guest room bed. But, wait. I have to put on the brakes. I simply cannot entertain as I have in the past.

While searching the closet for clean guest towels, I run across the plastic sacks of silk flowers. What am I going to do with them? I don't know how to put these together for my hats, and I don't feel up to a project that requires a lot of learning.

It's late in the afternoon when Walt and Barb pull into our driveway. For dinner, we order a pizza, which feels to me like a major defeat, as I would have preferred to prepare a feast. But this isn't a war or even a contest; it's relatives here for a nice weekend.

While we wait for the pizza, Jim sets out crackers and cheese and pickled herring and a bottle of zinfandel. After a few sips of wine, I'm dizzy. Since the start of chemo, alcohol seems more potent. The 12 percent ethanol in wine hits me as if it has grown to 80 proof. In my wine-soaked muddle, I remember the flowers.

"Barb," I say, dangling a sack in each hand, "do you know anything about making corsages out of silk flowers?"

"Let me see those." Barb dumps the white, burgundy, cornflower-blue, and lemon-yellow blooms onto the dining room table and goes to work. One by one she inspects the blossoms, twists their wire stems, and turns their fabric leaves. "How's that?" she mutters to herself as she places the sprigs against the brims of my hats. Looking up, she says, "We need florist's wire and ribbon and green tape."

"Walt and Jim," she calls to our husbands, "let's go to the silk flower store."

Barb spends the next two days at the dining room table, snipping blooms, tearing off excess silk leaves, fashioning bows from ribbon, tying the stems together with florist's tape. She hums as she works and examines each cluster of flowers at arm's length to get the longer view. She secures each corsage, one after the other, to the brims of my hats with milliner's pins and says, "Here, try this on. Let's see if that works."

They're truly stunning, absolutely gorgeous. I now have at least twenty corsages of various sizes and colors to match every piece of clothing I own.

Recently I haven't laughed as much as I used to. While Barb and Walt are here, however, Jim cooks and we laugh. It feels so good to tip my head back, open my mouth wide, and let the joy tumble out. Our friends Sally and Bill invite the four of us to dinner and we laugh. Wondrous moments erupt like champagne bubbles and we laugh.

What's so funny?

- Walt learning to cast a fly rod across our backyard.
- Sore back jokes. We kill a bottle of bourbon trying to cure all the bad backs in the house.
- The jelly beans and chocolate eggs that we eat from last week's Easter basket.
- The case of grapefruit that arrives at our house every month from someone named Red Cooper. Jim thought he had

ordered one shipment, and four years later we are still getting grapefruit.

- The mallards, now a committed threesome of two males and one female, beside our pond. Walt names them Huey, Dewey, and Louise.
- The eighteen years of wine bottle corks I have saved.
- The "bump out," my proposed addition to our bedroom that would add eight feet of floor space to the east, two walls of windows, and a fireplace. Jim thinks this is the stupidest idea he has ever heard.

We take a trip to the rare-wood sawmill and buy breadboards. We drive past my favorite house in Ann Arbor, a stone cottage tucked into a copse of oaks and pines. We eat Great Harvest cinnamon rolls for breakfast. We watch cowbirds at the feeders and a flock of cedar waxwings in the cherry tree. I'm absolutely thrilled, absolutely exhausted.

A dream: I watch handless fingers typing the words *somewhat* and *including,* over and over, on a computer keyboard. What's going on in my head to produce these images? The *somewhat* is easy; it describes the tentativeness that rules my life right now. And the *including*? Maybe it refers to a hope, a wish that a cosmic force will wrap itself around me and draw me into a larger, pleasurable universe crowded with my friends.

The shower spray beats against my body as I'm preparing to go to work. I rub a dollop of shampoo into my hair. A wad of loose strands comes off in my hand. Same thing happens with the dollop of creme rinse. By the end of the shower, I've made five hair balls, each about a half inch in diameter.

It's happening. The dreaded event is here. I call Jane and arrange for a pixie haircut tomorrow noon.

"Look what I found." Jane reaches into her cabinet and pulls out what looks like a dead raccoon. She gives it a shake, and the pile of animal fur becomes a wig. "I spotted it at a beauty supply shop last week and thought, 'That will be perfect for Janet.' And, it's only thirty-four dollars."

The floor of her hairdresser's bay is littered with my hair. All that she has left on my scalp is a bang across my forehead, a fringe that tickles the top of my neck, and short, thick stubble in between. Jane sets the wig on my head. She tucks and snips and twists the plastic locks. She's right. It *does* look like my previous hairdo.

I hate the pixie cut. Jim marvels at how good it looks, and I think it's awful.

Bill, Sally, Jim, and I go to a Wynton Marsalis "dance party" at the Eastern Michigan University gymnasium. I wish I had a bag over my head because I look ridiculous with short hair. Bill and Sally admire it. They're being kind.

While out on the gym floor trying to learn a few steps of a funky dance, I notice a big shot from the university staring at me from across the room. He's probably trying to figure out who this familiar-looking, but not quite right, person is. I avoid his stare. I don't want to acknowledge him.

I give up on learning the dance steps and sit in the bleachers. Suddenly, I'm smothered by the presence of the other people in the gym. They close in from all sides; their proximity is strangling me. They are breathing their germs out into the air, and I, with a white blood cell count that is undoubtedly way too low, am breathing them in. They cough. They sneeze. As they dance, the germy clouds that surround each of them break loose and drift my way. It's dangerous for me to be here. I came to the dance party because I forgot that I'm not normal, that I'm vulnerable. I want to race to the car, want to escape the microbial threat.

This morning in the shower, my hair comes out by the handfuls and clogs the bathtub drain. Blond commas carpet the tiled floor and dot the shoulders of my black linen jacket. I slip a clump of hair into an envelope and bury it in the bottom of my jewelry drawer. Maybe in the future I'll want to remember what my real hair was like.

My scalp is very tender, feels as if someone has yanked each hair out one by one. I notice it mostly at night when I turn my head and the remaining short hairs brush against the pillow. I don't understand why my skull feels like a patch of boils. Jane says each hair has a little muscle that anchors it to my scalp, and after being tortured by the chemo, those muscles have cramps.

Now the lady in the mirror has no hair. The ridges along the tops of her orbits are bare, and the edges of her eyelids—without lashes— look like smooth, rubber crescents. If I avoid the mirror, I can pretend my hairless twin doesn't exist.

I discover that a hat on a bald head looks dorky, like an inadequate hat plopped on top of an obviously bald head. It needs something to fill in the borders where hair usually grows, to occupy the empty spaces around my ears and at the nape of my neck. My answer is head scarves. I tie a scarf, selected to match my clothes as well as the flowers on that day's hat, around my bare head and leave the scarf tails to hang artfully down the back of my jacket. At least I hope it appears artful. That's my goal.

At night, my bald head gets cold, so I wear the cotton knit snuggy cap I ordered from the American Cancer Society catalog. Around the house, I either wear just a scarf or go bare. Sometimes, when I'm in a hurry, I start out the backdoor with nothing on my head. The cool air against my scalp reminds me I need a covering. What if, as the weather warms up, I drive all the way to work or to the grocery store or to the bookshop and find I'm not wearing a hat? As an insurance policy I stash a spare scarf and denim cloche, a yellow sunflower pinned to its brim, in the backseat of my car.

Samya, one of the pediatric doctors, is Muslim and wears her hair covered at all times. We talk about the wearing of the scarf. For her, it represents adherence to the tenets of her faith; for me, it represents the loss of something I treasured more than I ever realized.

Some people say the most unhelpful things, such as "You're so lucky that the chemo can cure the cancer." Or "Sinead O'Connor [a singer who took a razor to her head] looks smashing." Or "My aunt/sister/cousin/mother/friend had breast cancer and her hair came in thick and curly." These bromides irritate me to my toes. I don't feel the least bit lucky. I'm not a star like Sinead O'Connor, and I didn't shave my head; I'm not young; I'm not Irish. I don't care what happened to someone else's aunt/sister/cousin/mother/friend. What has happened to me is overwhelming and terrible.

Jane the miracle-making hairdresser and Amy at work tell me I have "good bones" for wearing hats. My facial features gene came from my father, passed down from his mother. Grandma Reed had high cheekbones; a tall, thin neck; and deep, mysterious eyes. When I look at pictures of Grandma, who never smiled when being photographed, I see the resemblance.

On the way to work this morning, sporting my purple-and-cream-colored scarf topped by my navy blue straw hat with a huge bouquet of silk lilacs pinned to the brim, I stop the car for a red light. A Lincoln Continental pulls to a halt beside me, and the two ladies inside point their fingers in my direction. One flashes a big smile and nods. Her hands gesture toward her head, and her lips motion the words "Great hat." In return, I smile and nod and answer, "Thanks."

A dream: I'm at a pediatric infectious diseases convention. I leave my hotel room and ride the elevator, a brass box lined with mirrors and lights and burgundy carpeting, to the lobby. I stride through the crowded registration area and suddenly realize I'm exposed. No scarf, no hat, no knit snuggy, only my nearly bald head sprouting the golden halo of fine hairs that makes me look like a newborn ostrich.

I'm horrified. It's the heart-stopping horror of an exposure dream, a being-in-public-while-naked dream, a taking-a-final-exam-when-you-forgot-to-go-to-class-all-semester dream. I race for the safety of my room. On the elevator going up, I realize that, although many people had *seen* me, no one has *recognized* me. It's a new type of security.

The wig is great to have, but I don't wear it often. It's hot and itchy and makes me feel phony. It's my Barbie Doll hair: stiff, plastic, and too much of it.

I do, however, wear the wig occasionally to work. Not when I'm sitting at the computer or reading or writing or talking on the phone in my office or meeting with my lab crew or the Pediatric Infectious Diseases clinical team. I wear it when I don't want to appear weak, such as when I meet with the dean and the executive committee of the medical school or during the Pediatric Infectious Diseases division budget meeting with the chairman of our department or when seeing old patients in the clinic.

I'm not doing any inpatient consultations while undergoing chemotherapy. The clinical service is too unpredictable. We may get from zero to seven new consultations a day. The infectious diseases fellows do a lot of the footwork in evaluating these patients, but, since I'm responsible for the final decisions, I need, as I have always done, to take a medical history, conduct a physical examination, review the laboratory work, and look at the x-rays. For the first week after chemo I absolutely can't do any of that, but during the two weeks before the next infusion, I might be able to manage zero to two patients a day, but no more. So I let my colleagues handle the inpatient consultations.

In addition, my white blood cell count is dangerously low. My oncologist decreased the doses of the Adriamycin and Cytoxan for my second infusion because my counts were so terrible after the first. As the infectious diseases doctor, if I were to see inpatients, I would take care of children, many of them with cancer and low blood counts themselves, who are infected with strange, hard-to-treat, awful bacteria, viruses, and fungi.

I imagine myself standing in the ICU with microscopic, deadly *Stenotrophomonas* and methicillin-resistant *Staphylococcus aureus* and vancomycin-resistant enterococci swarming on every surface. I don't want to place myself at risk of becoming infected with those germs. Even though I wash my hands between every patient—and have the crusty skin to prove it—I don't want to take any chances.

One of my long-term patients—I have taken care of her for at least eight years—is scheduled to see me this morning in the clinic. Her mother is smart, meticulously well groomed, demanding, manipulative, and coy—a very forceful advocate for her chronically ill daughter. I like Mrs. R.'s spunk and always look forward to seeing her and Rebecca. She likes me, too, because I listen to her requests and her endless questions and I agree that her daughter's life, limited as it is, has great value.

Wearing my wig, I stroll into the examining room as if this visit is no different from any other.

"Good morning. How are things going with you and Becky?" I say to Mrs. R's back. She is adjusting her daughter in the wheelchair.

She turns toward me, raises her hands to her face, opens her eyes wide in horror, and groans, "Oh, no, Dr. Gilsdorf. OH, NO." She wraps her arms around me and gasps, "Are you OK?"

"Yes, I'm OK," I answer.

Mrs. R. probably wants more details about why I have lost weight, look gaunt, and wear a wig. She has depended on me for nearly a decade. She knows her daughter will die sooner rather than later—we have talked about that, planned for that. But she's not prepared for me to go away. She must feel blindsided and soon to be abandoned.

"I'm definitely going to be OK," I say gently. I need to reassure Mrs. R. I don't want to add the question of my well-being to her already heavy burden.

We aren't here, however, to discuss my health but, rather, to discuss Becky's health. I want to be sure our focus remains on the business at hand, on the reason they come to see me every three to four months, on what is best for her daughter.

"Now, how's Becky?" I ask.

A dream: I'm responsible for the care of a sixteen-year-old patient who has osteomyelitis, an infection in his leg bone. He is kept in a Frisbeesized, disc-shaped metal container that looks like a ten inches in diameter flying saucer suspended by a chain from the hospital ceiling. Daily, the resident physicians-in-training report on his status, and, daily, I say, "You're nuts. There's no patient in that metal disc."

"Oh, yes, there is," they reply and detail his intravenous antibiotic infusions, his vital signs, his laboratory results, the progress of his infection.

I continue to disbelieve them but never check the contents of the metal disc myself. Why? Am I an incompetent physician? Fearful? Avoiding a difficult situation? Where does the dream end and reality begin?

The alopecia from Adriamycin is total. No scalp hair, no eyebrows, no eyelashes. My nose runs all the time, so I keep a folded tissue in every pocket of everything I wear. I finally figure out that my nose constantly drips mucus because my eyes constantly drip tears, which is a reaction to irritants that my eyelashes used to filter out. I've tried to draw new eyebrows with the pencil from the "Look Good, Feel Better" kit, but I end up resembling a manikin.

Besides no head hair, alopecia means no pubic hair. The husband of a woman I know who had cancer said making love was like having sex with a nine-year-old.

At Busch's supermarket the man ahead of me in the checkout line looks like Robert Redford dressed as a lumberjack. His complexion is ruddy but healthy, he wears a green plaid flannel shirt, and his sandy hair sticks out from his scalp as if he just crawled out of bed.

I look past him and stare at the cranberry juice display, at the pyramid of jugs filled with red liquid. They remind me of Adriamycin, and, reminiscent of Pavlov's dogs, my stomach starts to churn. As I squirm, I tug at the scarf under my straw hat, rearranging its folds, straightening its knot. I don't notice that the line is moving. I don't hear the checkout guy in the next lane say to me, "I'll take you over here." The lumberjack man turns and waves me forward, saying, "Ma'am . . ."

I nod a thank you to him and say, "I guess I'm a little distracted today."

He flashes a kind, knowing smile and says, "I understand. I paid my dues about seventeen years ago."

Those words, loaded with acceptance and understanding from a stranger, tell a strong story. They speak of our exclusive club. Even though I undoubtedly will never meet the lumberjack man again, I feel close to him, as he and I are charter members. Unlike people who belong to golf or tennis or sailing clubs, the members of our club are bound by golden filaments that know no status, have no monetary value, depend on no fancy clothes or expensive sports gear or the latest electronic equipment or expensive booze. We are tied together by the hard-earned knowledge of what matters most in life.

In my journal I write:

> *Good things about chemo . . .*
> • *Weight loss (will it stay off?)*
> • *Don't have to shave legs*
> • *Don't have to tweeze whiskers off chin*
> • *Don't have to wash hair and blow dry*
> *Bad things about chemo . . .*
> *EVERYTHING ELSE!*

# Chapter 13

Seeing Purple Seashells and
Other Unexpected Things

In my journal I write:

*What's real? What's imagined? This is like living an inside-out
dream. If I could awaken from the nightmare of reality, then I
could fall into the peace of no arm pain, no nausea.*

There's rhythm to chemotherapy: infusion on Friday; sleep and feel
like vomiting all weekend; wander apathetically around the house on
Monday and Tuesday; drive to the store for the *New York Times* and
check the office e-mail from home on Wednesday; take a walk in
Parker Mill Park or the University Botanical Gardens on Thursday;
work at the computer from home on Friday. During weeks two and
three, I go to my office for four or five hours and come home for a nap.
Over and over. The synchrony gives structure, albeit warped, to my
new life. It keeps me connected, if only by a thread, to my real life.

A new aspect of the routine is baths—long, leisurely soaks in
warm, soothing water. A scoop of perfumed salts adds a hint of flair
where otherwise there is none.

I don't read in the tub. Rather, I lie on my back with a towel folded
behind my neck, adjust the faucet with my toes, and let the ripples lap
my ears. I'm here to relax, to hand over my restlessness and worries
and ragged nerves to the therapeutic water. But, soon my brain begins
to flit from thought to thought like an anxious wren, searching for a
challenging idea, one that's doable within my current limits. My limbs

itch to go—anywhere. Lounging in this bathtub feels like a colossal waste of time, but, boy, do I have lots of time.

Back in my real life, the one that seems a million years ago, I planned, scheduled, arranged, and strategized to maximize my productivity. Now, reverse scheduling guides my days. I string tasks along, one . . . then another . . . then another, to occupy the endless hours. I play solitaire. I look at pictures in decorating magazines. I take leisurely baths.

In my journal I write:

*Time is a burden, an empty vessel to be filled with simple activities so, when full, it will pass faster.*

I reread the passage I just wrote, and it doesn't make sense. An empty vessel is a burden? What's full? the vessel? the burden? time? What's "it"? activities? the vessel? time? Which state of mind is the most accurate, that of the writer (me) or of the reader (me)?

It's called "chemo brain," and it's very real, as my oncologist warned before my treatment began. "Women whose work requires a high degree of cognitive activity sometimes find, during chemotherapy, they can't think as well as before," he said. "You may experience this, too."

During my laboratory's research meeting, nearly two weeks after a chemo infusion, I fidget. I cross my left leg over my right and then back again. I pick at a paper clip. I draw figure eights on the table with my pencil eraser. One after the other, around the table, the students and postdocs and technicians each describe their work during the past week. They leave me in the intellectual dark. I can't concentrate on what they're saying. As one finishes speaking and the next begins, I'm left to wonder, "Now, why were we doing this experiment in the first place?" "Which antibody are you using, again?" "What marker, protein, plasmid, gene are you talking about?" The facts bombard me too rapidly; my understanding dawns too slowly. The concepts are deep, and I can't remember the context that gives meaning to the data. I'm afloat, ungrounded, as if I just spent five minutes in Paris, then five minutes in Istanbul, then Venice, Oslo, Jerusalem, Madrid.

Undoubtedly my lab team realizes I'm not the same as before, but they don't mention it. Rather, they pretend nothing has changed. They're showing me the highest respect. Carl is very gentle when he corrects an error in my thinking in front of the whole group. Will it ever come back? Will I ever be able to effectively lead my laboratory again?

I'm even hesitant with knitting and don't feel capable of starting a new sweater, particularly one that I design myself. I have no novel pattern ideas, no tenacity to translate an idea into a method or a method into a completed, well-constructed garment. I worry that, in the end, I will fail, that when the sweater is finished I'll hate it, ball it up, and throw it in the trash. So I make dishrags, little eight-by-eight-inch squares knit on big, size 7 needles, reassured that if I make a mistake, it won't matter. Nobody cares about imperfect dishrags.

In my writing—my cherished writing—I'm crippled by memory gaps, by surface thinking and an inability to probe the depths of an idea, by word blank-outs that are different from the age-related absences I've had since before chemo. During the old-style lapses, no matter how long I stall on a word, I cannot retrieve it, until maybe a week later. Now, during the new-style lapses, if I pause and imagine the word written on the computer screen, similar to the news streamers that crawl across the TVs at the airport, I can usually see that projected word and capture it.

During the weekend following each chemo infusion I can't read anything. Then, over the next week, I begin to handle the *New York Times,* at least the first third of moderate-sized articles. The *Ann Arbor News* is, for the most part, better. Crossword puzzles are impossible, as is reading the emotion-laden stories in the *Sun. House Beautiful, Elle Décor, House and Garden* are full of pictures, so I absentmindedly turn the pages, studying the draperies, bedspreads, kitchen cupboards, and bathroom wallpaper.

This is the rhythm of my days.

Not only am I "experiencing chemo brain," as my oncologist predicted, but I'm participating in a School of Nursing study to quantify the magnitude of my disordered thinking. The first measurements, taken immediately after beginning my chemotherapy, will be compared to those obtained at various times over the next four months. These tests will document recall and spacial perception and endurance.

The study coordinator has me recite from memory increasingly long strings of numbers.

"7, 3, 6, 9, 1," she says.

"7, 3, 6, 9, 1," I answer. A list of this length is easy, as it echoes the rhythm of the five-digit intrauniversity phone numbers.

When she gets to nine numbers, I stumble.

"2, 6, 3, 1, 9, 5, 8, 4, 7," she says.

"2, 6, 3, 1 . . . I can't remember, maybe 8 or 4? . . . I give up."

"OK," she says, "now I'll recite a series of numbers and you repeat them backwards."

Ugh, I think. This is going to be gruesome.

"8, 4, 7," she says.

"7, 4, 8," I answer.

When she gets to five digits, I bail out.

"4, 7, 3, 6, 1," she says.

"1 . . . Um, I know the first number was 4, so the last one in my answer would be 4. Beyond that, I'm stumped."

This exercise in memory frustrates me, because, ordinarily, I like to win—at games, at contests, at solitaire, at getting grants funded, at diagnostic challenges. Now, although my competitive spirit is still alive, my oomph for sustained work isn't.

Next she has me recall, after five minutes and again after thirty minutes, associations between random words and nonsense figures. This is a little easier than the numbers, because I can invent fanciful associations, such that "plate" and ⊣| go together because the figure can be seen as one plate on end, preceded by two mirror-image bent saucers.

Next she times the speed at which I serially connect the numbered dots. The secret to success is to always look ahead, to search for the next number while my pencil is moving toward the previous one.

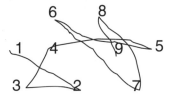

Then she projects a three-dimensional stick box on a computer screen. I'm supposed to push the "enter" button each time the front-to-back orientation of the box changes.

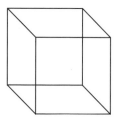

Staring at the hollow cube makes me dizzy, and I don't understand how it works. This could be a hoax. Does the orientation really change, or is it an optical illusion? I hit "enter" several times but am not sure if I blinked or if the image actually flipped.

Over the weeks of the study, my accumulated dose of chemo increases but my performance on her tests stays the same. *I* think she's not measuring the right things. My deficits, while absolute, are more subtle than what she can detect. Is my brain problem really a physiologic effect of the drugs, or does it reflect a psychic reaction to—and shutdown from—my life being turned completely upside down? Doesn't matter. Regardless of the pathophysiology, my mind just doesn't work right.

A dream: I see a confluence of global trade and food safety. These issues, each vague, are separated by a huge expanse, as if they were balanced on the ends of the biggest teeter-totter in the universe. Slowly they move toward each other until they converge like the marriage of two swarms of bees. The dilemma in the dream becomes clear: how to safely transfer leftovers from shiny, oak tables in wealthy American dining rooms to mats on mud floors in impoverished African huts. The images march through my sleeping brain like railroad cars—little stacks of fresh pineapple cubes, little piles of cherry-walnut scones. This may be a wish dream, one about being able to taste food, except that, in reality, I don't like pineapple.

$$\text{\it※}$$

The reviewers' comments and the editorial decision from *Infection and Immunity*—to publish my manuscript or to reject it—have finally arrived. I glance at the first sentence in the editor's letter. It says, "Your paper, entitled 'Comparative analysis of the pilus adhesins of *H. influenzae* biotype IV strains,' does not meet the criteria for publication in *Infection and Immunity*."

Rejected. Another failure. I know this research isn't destined for a Nobel prize, but it's an interesting observation and the science is solid. To me, when I submitted this paper for review, *Infection and Immunity* seemed to be a good home for it.

I worked hard on this manuscript and wrote it through the lens of "chemo brain," so my ability to concentrate and to follow a line of reasoning over the hills and into the valleys of the experiments was compromised. Still, I thought I did the job well.

I can't face this, can't bear to read the whole letter, so I toss it back into my wire in-basket.

It's been a week since the reviews and editor's decision arrived, and I haven't had the stomach to look at them again. Yesterday I moved them from the bottom of the in-basket to a pile of other papers on my office floor but still couldn't face reading them.

This is silly, I tell myself. Grow up. Accept defeat gracefully. Hold your head high with pride even though your ego is in tatters. I sift through the papers on the floor, file the ones that need to be filed and throw away the rest, except for the dreaded correspondence from *Infection and Immunity*. It remains on my lap, spread across the fabric of my linen pants. In a burst of daring, I pick it up, slide the pages from the envelope, and force myself to read the reviewers' comments.

Their suggestions are minor: delete one redundant figure, clarify a section the reviewer didn't understand. So why did the editor reject the paper?

I reread the editor's letter, a form letter; this time I read it through to the end. The second paragraph gives instructions for resubmitting the manuscript after I have addressed the concerns of the reviewers. I read the letter yet again. The editor didn't reject the paper after all; he just didn't accept it as originally written and wants a revision.

This letter—not a rejection and, in the end, not a problem—hovered like a storm cloud over my head for a week. Such is my current place in the world. I'm tired of competing, tired of being rejected, just plain tired.

There's a four-harness floor loom in the corner of the Cancer Center's blood-drawing station. Does anyone actually weave while they wait? How many people who come here even know how to make a shed and then work a shuttle through it? Apparently not many, for only six inches of weft is twined through the warp, the same as when I first started coming for blood tests.

"Card, please," the clerk says.

I pull my patient card from the plastic pocket that hangs around my neck—from behind my hospital employee ID badge and my buy-ten-get-one-free coffee ticket—and hand it to her.

"Have a seat," she says. I don't feel like weaving this morning so I choose a chair far from the loom and begin thumbing through an old travel magazine.

A hospital volunteer pushes her refreshment cart toward me. She smiles sweetly and says, "Would you like tea or coffee or . . . ?" In midsentence, she eyes my hospital ID badge, jerks her cart back, and says, "Uh . . . no." Her glossed lips frown, her penciled eyebrows purse, and her lids, thick with mascara, narrow. "Are you a hospital employee?"

"Well, yes, I am," I say. "And I'm also a patient."

"Oh, OK." She pushes the cart back toward me. "Coffee?" she asks again.

I'm appalled. Does she really think hospital employees sit around the blood-drawing station and pilfer the patients' refreshments? Did she fail to notice that this hospital employee has no hair?

"No," I answer. I don't want her coffee. It's contaminated with pettiness.

✿

This seems to be a good year for birds—"dickie birds," as Jim calls them—in our backyard. A goldfinch, yellow as butter, flies off his perch on the thistle-filled feeder when a second goldfinch comes in for a landing; when a third goldfinch arrives, the second flies off in an avian do-si-do. At the mixed seed feeders, a caste system seems to dictate who eats when. The house finches, their ruby heads bobbing at the seeds, scatter when the squawking blue jay nears, who then leaves when a coal-colored crow swoops in.

Cardinals rocket across the yard from treetop to treetop, the red of their bodies like flames against the backdrop of green leaves. As the mourning doves strut on the porch railing, their colors turn from muddy water to half-strength tea to caramel to saddle soap with each waddling step. Nuthatches, head down and tail up, peck bugs from the beech bark, and a hummingbird hovers like a tiny helicopter at a petunia bloom. In a blink, he flits ten feet leftward to hover at a bloom on the trumpet vine.

This is theater—the theater of the birds—and it entertains me on clear, sunny, lazy afternoons on my back porch. I like the simplicity of the birds, the beauty of their movements, the melodies of their gossip.

✿

On the Thursday before Memorial Day, another theater—the theater of America—plays at the Rite Aid drugstore. A black woman, tall and straight, her fist gripping a ring of keys, and her lanky teenage son wearing yellow sunglasses that wrap around his face rearrange the Pepsi display. They pull six two-liter plastic bottles of Vernors soda from the middle of the stack and set them in their shopping cart beside four bags of potato chips. Leaving the Pepsi pyramid, the son says to his mother, "Now we need a Michigan flag."

A middle-aged, curly-haired woman approaches the cash register with a box of mulberry-colored bath soaps, each shaped like a seashell.

"Four dollars and thirty-seven cents," the clerk, an octogenarian whose name tag reads "LUIS," tells her.

She sets four one-dollar bills and a handful of change on the counter. The woman's words, seemingly French, are uninterpretable. Luis doesn't know what to do. He glares at her. His white eyebrows knit into a question. Bewildered, she turns to the person behind her in line, a young mother whose toddler wrestles to escape her arms. The young mother adjusts the squirming child on her hip, steps to the counter, sets her hand on the money, and pushes two quarters toward Luis.

"She needs change," the mother says.

They are vibrant, these characters that were once invisible to me. Now they loom large and lovely and important against the store's backdrop of magazines, candy bars, cosmetics, and clocks. In scenes that would have been mundane six months ago, these people are preparing, sharing, helping, living.

✦

A dream: Jim calls to somewhere in South Carolina and ends up talking with a sergeant whose name is Kevin Kevin, a supposed high school friend of Joe's. Handing me the phone, Jim returns to connecting a new laser printer to our computer. Kevin Kevin and I chat about the military and Joe and old times, and I'm impressed by his persistent immaturity. Finally—by this time I'm sitting in the maintenance bay of a car repair place and Kevin Kevin has turned into an old boyfriend of mine—I say to him, "Kevin, you should know what else is going on here. . . . I have breast cancer." In the space of five fleeting dream seconds, thirty years unfolded while spinning through an Alice in Wonderland cosmos.

Until my cancer, I hadn't taken a nap since I was two years old. Cat has now taught me how to nap. Curled into a furry O, she likes to lie on my pillow beside my face.

In the half dawn of waking, I hear my heartbeat reflected through the mattress. It gallops at about two hundred beats per minute.

"Now what?" I say out loud, my brain crawling out of sleep. My heart's too fast. Why? What would make my heart race like this? Cardiomyopathy? Has my heart turned into a flabby mass that quivers rather than beats? A heart that can't pump with enough vigor to get my blood out to my capillaries? Cardiomyopathy is one of the side effects of the Adriamycin.

I sit up and take my pulse. It's normal. I lie back down.

My heartbeat is galloping again. Once more I sit up and take my pulse, in my left wrist, my right wrist, and the carotid arteries in my neck. They're all normal.

By now I'm completely awake. Cat continues to doze on my pillow. The rapid pulse . . . the sleeping cat. I nod with understanding. The racing heart belongs to her.

A dream: I live in a women's cooperative. Our communal vehicle, which I drive from time to time, is named the Female Mobile. It consists of an upholstered seat, covered in lush, plum-colored velvet, mounted at a slightly backwards tilt on an automobile chassis. It has no sides, no roof. It also has no steering wheel, but I maneuver the car through the university parking garage by simply leaning my body in the direction I want to go. I'm motoring, without effort, without restraint, as free of baggage as a sheikh on a flying carpet.

I've seen her in the bookstore often, the young clerk with a pleasant, pretty face. Lazy curls brush the tops of her ears; thin, wire-rimmed glasses perch on her nose. She walks with a serious, unhurried air. And her arm is impossible to miss, the short, twisted right arm that swings uselessly at her side.

Today she wears a loose summer dress with a neckline that dives four inches down her breastbone. Peeking above the fabric is a scar, a well-healed, silvery pink sternotomy scar. This glimpse of her chest completes her story for me. While still a child, maybe even as a baby, she had cardiac surgery. As a complication of her surgery, or possibly of the heart disease that required the operation, she had a stroke that paralyzed her right arm.

And she's pregnant. A round, firm basketball of about seven months' gestation protrudes under her dress. As she moves toward the cash register, her body glides with confidence that she is adored, that her lover doesn't care about her chest scar or her gimpy arm, that their baby won't, either.

Later in the afternoon, I stop the car for a red light in downtown Ann Arbor. A man and a woman stand on the sidewalk, talking, in the glare of the midday sun. He is stiff and formal, trussed up in a business suit. She, red-headed and laughing, holds open the door to a building. On her left thigh, a square patch of pale skin runs for three inches below the cuff of her shorts. It's fairly fresh, this skin donor site. Where was the harvested skin grafted to? Her legs are tanned and otherwise unblemished. Her arms, moving with the ease of a breeze as she speaks, are flawless. Her face is freckled, its features intact. The graft must be under her clothes. The man's eyes are drilled on her as if the rest of the world has evaporated. He grins at her laughter.

Near the gift shop in the children's hospital, the serious, principled face of a seven-year-old mirrors that of the woman, obviously her mom, beside her. They walk around the corner in synchrony, their pigeon-toed gaits identical, the swing of their hips identical. A dad-the-horse, his ears cupped by the pudgy thighs of a four-year-old, trots down the hall with his son on his shoulders. A three-year-old, pushing his stroller, steers it into the wall; his mother winces at the impact and redirects the stroller.

Where have they been all this time, these normal people who go about their normal lives while housed in abnormal bodies? Who share with their kids their own unique talents and interests and creative solutions to life's challenges? Who, in everyday obscurity, live out their love of vintage cars or bass fishing; their passion for singing in a church choir; their flair for blue fingernail polish or turtle figurines; their ability to play the saxophone, to plant a peony bush, to make a quilt or homemade lemon bars or a wooden truck?

How about the classic Craftsman detail on the house near Dixboro Road that I notice for the first time on the way home? The lime-green leaves on the maple tree in front of the old school? The pump and grave marker and "RR Xing" sign in Evelyn's yard? Have they been behind a drape, a thick, translucent drape?

# CHAPTER 14

Iatrogenesis

*Iatrogenesis: disease "induced unintentionally by a physician through his diagnosis, manner, or treatment; of or pertaining to the induction of (mental or bodily) disorders, symptoms, etc., in this way."* —*Oxford English Dictionary*, 2d edition, online

My oncologist is out of town this week; he told me at the last visit that his physician assistant (PA) would see me in the clinic today before my infusion. That's OK, as all doctors, even mine, need a vacation from their patients every once in a while.

My first stop is the blood-drawing station. I extend my right arm; no tourniquets or blood pressure cuffs or injections are allowed in my bad left arm. The phlebotomist chatters pleasantly as he ties the elastic band below my shoulder and taps the vein in my antecubital fossa. Easily, almost painlessly, he slips the needle into the vein in the bend of my elbow and fills two tubes with my blood. The sample goes immediately to the lab for my preinfusion blood counts.

Next stop is the examining room in the oncology clinic, where I try to read as I wait. My attention drifts from the front page of my newspaper to the vein on my right hand where, later, Alice will start my IV. The skin, bloodless and pallid, looks dead. Even though it's summer outside, a winterlike glare from the fluorescent bulbs overhead stains the walls, the paper covering the examining table, the Formica counter—everything in here, including me—a faint cobalt blue. It's cold. The ventilating system is blowing chilly air.

I dread what's ahead this weekend, the queasy misery that will tie me to both my bed and the orange mixing bowl, will turn my muscles to mush, will fog my brain, will churn my guts for the next three days. Since yesterday I've ingested only lemonade and water in the hope that I will get through tonight without vomiting.

The door eases open, and the PA steps in. I refold the *New York Times*, trapping the world's mayhem between its pages, and set it on my pile of clothes.

"We have a problem," she says.

My body tightens. Now what, I wonder. What could be wrong?

"Your counts are very low. Too low to get your chemo today."

"What are they?"

"Your white count is 2 and your ANC is 700."

That *is* low; I have only 700 neutrophils in every milliliter of my blood, whereas normally I should have more than 2,000. My risk of serious infection goes up with fewer than 1,000 and WAY up with fewer than 500. Another blast of chemo today will drive these counts down further.

"Actually," I explain, "they're the same as before my previous infusion."

My oncologist's words echo in my mind. "We take advantage of the cell cycling patterns when we plan the infusions," he explained before starting the chemo.

It's the dance of the M, G1, S, and G2 phases of all cells, including malignant ones, that determines my chemotherapy routine. The synchrony between the drugs and the cycles is important, because dosing the medicines too frequently or too far apart reduces their effectiveness. If I get the Adriamycin on schedule, by the time of the next infusion most of my cancer cells will be in the S phase, the stage at which this drug works best; if the infusion is delayed, if the cells have rolled through S phase into G2 phase or even into M phase, the drug won't kill them as well.

The regularity, the cadence, the pulse of the plan are mileposts on the road I travel. The rule is to step to the beat of the drum, stay the course. I *know* my doctor wouldn't want to delay my infusion.

"I think we should wait until next week," she says kindly.

"I'm not sure Dr. Miller would want to do that," I say, not so kindly. I really don't want to be a difficult patient, but I really don't want to miss my dose. Bad as the chemo is, not getting it today is worse.

"Dr. Gilsdorf," she says, acquiescing to my professional status, "you know the risks of neutropenia. We don't want to do anything that would hurt you."

I respect what she's saying. She doesn't want my ANC to get too low, doesn't want me to develop a serious infection. "But," I say, standing my ground, "you *need* to hurt me to get rid of my cancer. That's the whole point here."

"Let me check with one of the other oncologists." She scurries out the door.

Alone again in the blue-tinted examining room, too upset to read the newspaper, I fume over our little face-off. I wish Dr. Miller were here. I don't like to second-guess what he would do, but I don't want to delay my chemo.

In truth, waiting one week wouldn't be a huge deal; the cell cycles aren't *that* rigid. But what if something else happens to keep me from getting my infusion next week? I don't know what that might be, perhaps a tornado in Ann Arbor or a Michigan-wide power failure or a global shortage of chemotherapy drugs; we're not talking logic here. But, if an unexpected crisis happens in the next seven days, I would really be in trouble. I, the master of risk avoidance, want the infusion today.

Soon the PA returns. She has discussed the situation with the oncologist covering for Dr. Miller, and they have agreed to proceed with the infusion.

I breathe a large relief-laden sigh.

"But," she adds, "he suggests we start you on G-CSF."

G-CSF is granulocyte colony stimulating factor; the trade name is Neupogen. It's a growth promoter that jump-starts the bone marrow to pump out more granulocytes (i.e., neutrophils), the infection-fighting white blood cells. The Cancer Center pharmacist hands me a box of ten tiny vials, each containing one milliliter, about a quarter teaspoon, of G-CSF.

"One dose per vial. One vial per day," he says. "Don't waste it, because it costs $150.00 per dose." Holy Hannah, I think, that's $1,500.00 for a week and a half of G-CSF. If I were working at minimum wage, every dose would cost almost three times as much as I would earn each day. I would have to make $18.75 an hour to pay for one day of G-CSF and would have nothing left for food or rent or bus fare or my kids' shoes. Fortunately our insurance will cover the cost. What do people who have no health-care insurance do? Unless they're millionaires, they either go into medical debt—a bottomless hole from which they can never emerge—or stay neutropenic and hope to hell they don't get a bad infection. The pharmacist also gives me ten tuberculin syringes and a handful of individually wrapped alcohol wipes, which I carefully align in the sack with the box of G-CSF to protect the tiny, pricey little vials from breaking.

The G-CSF is given by subcutaneous injection. No one has shown me how to do that. I guess they figure a physician would know such a simple procedure. The truth is that I haven't *ever* been formally taught how to give an injection. That's a nursing activity.

My inexperience with injections doesn't worry me. Years ago as desperate interns at Ben Taub General, the county hospital in Houston, Texas, we did all kinds of things we hadn't been trained to do. When I, because all the clinic nurses had gone for the night, needed to give a child an injection of an antibiotic, I did what I had seen the nurses do and hoped I remembered it correctly.

Besides, I'm a seasoned self-venipuncturist. When I first established my research laboratory in Ann Arbor, we used my blood for the hemagglutination (HA) assays. Early one evening I wanted to set up an HA assay to incubate overnight so I could read the results first thing in the morning. I roamed the wards of the children's hospital searching for a resident physician to draw 10 cc of my blood for the assay but couldn't find anyone. Finally, impatient, hungry, and eager to go home, I said under my breath, "Forget it, I'll do it myself."

Alone in my laboratory, I tied a thick rubber band around my left upper arm, swabbed alcohol over my antecubital fossa, and jammed a butterfly needle into the large, blue vein at my elbow's crease. Forever after, I have drawn my own blood. Now that I have cancer, my lab crew teases me that the chemo will make my red blood cells goofy and, thus, ruin their experiments. They might be right. We currently use someone else's blood for the HA assays.

Although subQ injections (sticking the needle deep into the fatty layer beneath the skin) are technically different from venipunctures (sticking the needle into a vein), the concept of sticking a needle into myself is the same. There's something a bit anxiety provoking about autoinjection. It hints of self-abuse, of illicit, unchaste, prohibited activities. It's what drug addicts do to themselves.

My last chemo was only three days ago, so I'm still a little loopy, but it's time to give the first G-CSF injection. I stare at my thigh, riddled with cellulite, and see my grandmother's thigh. She lived in a tiny one-bedroom house in Morningside, Minnesota, the downscale, next-door neighbor to Edina, Minnesota, home to the wealthy. When I was a baby she developed diabetes and, for years, gave herself insulin. Every morning, before brewing coffee or making grandpa's oatmeal, she set a small enamel pan of water on her ancient gas stove and boiled a steel needle and a glass syringe. After they cooled, she filled the syringe with insulin from a little vial stored on the top shelf of her refrigerator.

Then she would sit at the dining room table, pull the hem of her seersucker housedress up to her crotch, unhook her stocking from its garter and roll it down, and swab alcohol on her pale but bruised, lumpy thigh—the one that looked then like mine does now. In one swift lunge, she stabbed the needle into her leg.

During visits to Minneapolis my sister Nancy and I would stand shoulder to shoulder in Grandma Nelson's dining room and, in absolute awe, hold our breath as she thrust her undoubtedly dull needle into herself.

"Doesn't that hurt?" we would whisper. We couldn't believe someone would, or could, do that.

"Naw," she always answered.

Now, I invert the vial as I have seen the nurses do, shove the needle through its rubber stopper, and pull on the plunger. The clear G-CSF, along with a little air, flows into the barrel of the syringe.

Pointing the needle at the ceiling, I push the plunger until the air is gone and a drop of G-CSF bubbles from the needle's tip.

I grab a thick fold of thigh with my left hand and rub an alcohol pad over the mound of cellulite that bulges into the V between my thumb and pointer finger. As I've seen many nurses do, I pull the plastic sleeve off the needle with my teeth. That may not be accepted technique, but it works. I take a deep breath, aim the needle at my leg, and ram it in.

Grandma Nelson was right. Sticking the needle—mine is twenty-five gauge, thin as a thread—into my leg doesn't hurt . . . much. I think it's about control. It would be worse if someone else were driving the needle. Pushing one milliliter of G-CSF into my tissue, though, hurts a little more, but not for long.

I'm the same age now as Grandma Nelson was when Nancy and I first watched the insulin shots. She's been dead for almost four decades, but this morning, the years seem to vanish and she's here with me, keeping me company, overseeing my hypodermic technique, giving me encouragement. The self-injection is a tactile echo through the generations: the pinch on the cellulite, the chill of icy alcohol, the prick of the needle, the sting of the medicine.

Medical and surgical therapies may have two effects, the intended one of healing and the unintended one of additional illness. The unwanted effects are intrinsic to good medical care, and even doctor-patients get them.

The faces of iatrogenesis are ugly. Complications of cancer therapy are irritating, expensive, and sometimes dangerous and include drug rashes, clots in leg veins from lying in bed too much, secondary cancers from immunosuppression and radiation, and parethesias and lymphedema from an axillary dissection. Sometimes they are layered one on top of another like the collapse of a house of cards; vomiting and neutropenia from chemo drugs may lead to dehydration and to bad infections. It's the rule of the wild—whatever my doctors do to me in the name of making me better may also make me sick.

My left leg itches. *Really* itches. Red bumps dot my kneecap. I decide to ignore it.

Two days later the rash has spread up and down that leg, over to the other leg, to one arm, and to my neck. Although I try not to touch it, apparently I scratch it during the night because the bumps are raised and some of the skin has been scraped off. This eruption might be from one of my drugs—in fact, I can't think of any other cause. It started three days after my chemo dose.

I call the Cancer Center and describe the itchy rash to the physician assistant. She agrees it might be from one of my medicines and suggests I watch it a little longer. Makes sense to me.

After two more days the rash continues to spread over both legs, both arms, and around my neck. It itches like hell. If I'm reacting to one of the drugs that was infused, it should be getting better by now. Maybe it's a reaction to the G-CSF, which I'm still taking.

I call the Cancer Center again.

"The rash is getting worse, and it's driving me absolutely nuts," I tell the physician assistant. "Besides, my husband and I were hoping to go up north, to Drummond Island, for a couple days. I'm reluctant to go so far away with this rash still spreading."

"I'll talk to Dr. Miller," she says.

Twenty minutes later she calls back. "Dr. Miller says to get yourself to the derm clinic as soon as you can. Could you make it before four o'clock? Dr. Avery will see you."

In less than an hour, I'm perched on the examining table in the dermatology clinic. I still feel crappy from the last dose of chemo, look like a hollow-eyed hag, and must appear ridiculous in my hat and scarf. My skin itches as if I've been bitten by ten thousand blackflies. I stare at my legs, at the ugly red bumps, at the purple-green bruises from scratching, at the places where I've clawed off the skin. I hate being a patient. I hate being in this clinic. I hate being ugly. I don't want to see yet another doctor who knows me in my real life, the me that went far, far away.

Dr. Avery examines the rash and asks questions. Any new soaps? New clothes? New lotions?

"None," I say. "I'm worried it might be the G-CSF or possibly one of the other drugs."

"Doesn't look like a drug eruption," he mutters, running his index finger over the bumps below my knee. "Looks more like contact dermatitis to me." He holds my hand and rotates my arm, checking the extent of the rash that runs from my right shoulder to my wrist.

"Well," he straightens up and says, "tell you what. If it's OK with Ben for you to have steroids, we'll give you a slow Medrol taper and see what happens."

I nod and my shoulders sag. I'm so tired of all this.

Coming home from the dermatology clinic, I turn the car into our driveway. Through the windshield the panorama of the front flower bed passes before me. Its border is clean. There are no grass heads bobbing above the day lilies, no thistles sprouting among the straw flowers. It's very satisfying, a clean flower bed, even though it took a lot of work to get that way.

"Aha," I say out loud as I drive into the garage. That's it. Mystery solved. Just before my last chemo dose I yanked a field of weeds from that flower bed. I remember kneeling on my left knee, the exact place where the rash started. The moisture from the ground soaked through the fabric of my pants, and I was mad about the grass and mud stains.

Ben approves of the steroids so I start taking the Medrol. Three days later the rash is a tiny bit better. At least it's no longer spreading. But there's a price for this improvement. Steroids make some people, including me, hyperactive.

I send an e-mail to the dermatologist.

```
From: Janet Gilsdorf
To: dermdoctor@umich.edu
Date: June 12, 2000 8:24:19 am
Subject: The rash
Rich, I figured out what caused the rash. You were
right, it's contact dermatitis. POISON IVY. I must
have kneeled in it while weeding the garden. The
```

steroids are helping some, but, BOY, am I wired.
Haven't slept for three nights. Thanks for your
help.
Janet


From: Richard Avery
To: janetgils@umich.edu
Date: June 12, 2000 11:49:56 AM
Subject: Re: The rash
Glad the rash is better. Hope you're being very
productive during your sleepless nights.
Rich

Jim's cereal bowl and spoon clink against the stainless steel of the kitchen sink. The heels of his boots clomp across the wooden floor. The backdoor opens and closes. He has gone to work and I'm still in bed, listening to *Morning Edition* and knitting dishrags.

A minute later, the back hall door opens and closes again, and the heels of Jim's boots clomp once more across the kitchen floor. He must have forgotten something.

Whap. A shiny, azure missile lands on the quilt beside me.

"Looks like they've finally started delivering it," Jim says. He has tossed the *New York Times,* wrapped in its signature blue plastic, to me. It's one of the best gifts imaginable. I won't have to keep four quarters in my pocketbook for the newspaper box or go to a store every day to buy one.

On top of everything else, now I have a sore tooth, the molar with the gold crown in my left lower jaw. It feels as if a popcorn husk or poppy seed is stuck between that tooth and the next. My left side seems to be jinxed.

For two days I dig at the tooth with my toothbrush, then a toothpick, then one of my hat pins. I floss morning and evening. Nothing comes loose. It continues to ache.

Now I'm worried it's an abscess. I imagine squiggly mouth bacteria twisted together in a pool of pus at the root of my tooth; never mind that I don't have enough white blood cells to make much pus. Even though it's Saturday I call my dentist. The message on his office's answering machine instructs me to phone him at home if this is an emergency. The message gives me his number, which neutralizes my guilt at phoning him on the weekend.

"Does it hurt more when you drink hot liquids?" he asks.

"No."

"Is it cold sensitive? Hurt when you drink cold liquids?"

"Yes."

"Is it pressure sensitive? Hurt when you bite down on something?"

"No."

He reassures me that these are the symptoms not of an infection but rather of nonbacterial irritation. He recommends Motrin, which I have already tried and which turns off the pain temporarily. He lists the possible causes of the pain: a slight change in alignment of the tooth or maybe bruxism. I reject the bruxism idea because at night I wear retainers, a leftover from orthodontia several years ago. They should keep me from grinding my teeth.

"I don't expect it to progress," he says. "It'll probably go away on its own. These things are usually pretty innocuous."

I tell one of Jim's neurosurgeon friends about the toothache and my attempts to treat it with a hat pin. Jason recommends the neurosurgeon's cure for pain: "You take a hammer and slam it on your thumb and the toothache will immediately vanish."

A week later, the examining room door in the oncology clinic tentatively opens. This time, rather than Ben or his physician assistant, a young man wearing a short, white clinical coat enters. He reaches for the toggle switch that alerts the staff to the status of the patient visit but flips the light switch instead. In a blink, the room is as dark as a coal mine.

I hear his hand groping the wall. Suddenly, light floods the room again. Oh, no, I think to myself. A medical student. I don't want to bother with a medical student, especially a fumbly one.

He introduces himself. His name tag reads "[Something] [Something], DDS."

"I see you're a dentist," I say.

He takes a seat at the desk, opens my file, and explains that he's completing an oral surgery residency, which includes a rotation in the oncology clinic. Surely, I conclude, he would rather see patients with cancers of the mouth and neck than of the breast.

So, it's balanced—he doesn't want to be here, and I don't want him here. This rotation, however, is required of him, and I'm being a good citizen. A multitude of patients allowed me to bungle through their care when I was in training, so I can tolerate a student every once in a while.

"How are you doing?" he asks.

"Actually, it's ironic. What's bothering me most right now is my sore tooth." I explain what my dentist said, tell him my orthodontist has checked my retainers and they aren't the cause of the pain.

"Let's take a look." By the beam of a penlight, he probes my mouth and taps my teeth with a tongue blade. He feels my neck, the angle of my jaw, the temporomandibular joint in front of my ear. He is confident, efficient, seems thrilled to be practicing dentistry again.

He concludes that I have bruxism. When I object, he says the retainers wouldn't prevent me from gnashing my teeth when I sleep.

"Why would I suddenly start bruxing?" I ask.

"Well," he says kindly, "you've been dealing with some pretty stressful stuff."

I shrug. I don't want to have a neurotic disease. Cancer is bad enough.

He says there's little to do for it other than positioning my tongue between my teeth to keep from grinding—while I sleep?—or using a tooth splint. On the way home I stop at the sporting goods store and buy a hockey mouth guard.

After my shower I rub a towel over my wet body, and a twinge of pain shoots through my left forearm. A red pimple has blossomed on my skin, halfway between my wrist and elbow.

Here it is, I think—my white blood cell count is below sea level, and the pimple is the start of an infection.

Ben had given me instructions for dealing with this. "Take ciprofloxacin at the first hint of an infection and then call me," he said.

There is no Cipro in our house so I phone in a prescription. It's Sunday morning and the neighborhood pharmacy hasn't opened yet. I leave an order on the answering machine. Only, I order levofloxacin instead of ciprofloxacin. Levo is a fairly new antibiotic and better than Cipro at treating the kinds of bacteria that cause skin infections.

Several hours later, the pharmacy has finally opened and the druggist has had time to fill my prescription. When I get home with the pills, I examine the pimple again. It hasn't changed a bit since early this morning. Maybe I don't need the antibiotic after all. I continue to watch the bump, and by the end of the day, it still hasn't changed. The levo goes into the medicine cabinet as insurance.

At my next oncology clinic appointment, I say, "Oh, Ben, I had an infection scare last week . . ."

"Did you start taking Cipro?"

"Well, no," I confess. "I called in a script for levo, and by the time it was filled, the little pimple hadn't changed so I didn't take it."

"Janet . . . Cipro." He leans forward and pats my arm. "I said to take Cipro."

"Yes, I know. But levo has better coverage for Gram-positive skin bugs."

"I said 'Cipro.'" He speaks slowly, emphatically, a cement wall of finality in his voice.

"OK." I'm defeated. "Next time I'll take Cipro."

At the beginning of my treatment I told Ben that *he* would be the doctor and *I* would be the patient. That was our agreement. Yet, infectious diseases is my specialty, and I know how to use antibiotics. What happened here is clear. Ben recommended Cipro because it has been studied extensively in cancer patients; current cancer practice guidelines suggest using ciprofloxacin for the initial treatment of infections. Yet, I know antibiotics. Levofloxacin would be better for cellulitis, which is what I would have been treating.

I'm not sure what I'll do next time I get a skin infection scare. Maybe it won't happen.

The side effects of the Taxol, which is the second phase of my chemotherapy, are different from those of Adriamycin and Cytoxan, the drugs from the first phase. Of note, two days have passed since my first Taxol infusion and I'm not nauseated at all. Everything still tastes like rusty nails, but there is no vomiting, no churning stomach, no spending the weekend in bed clutching the orange mixing bowl. This is a piece of cake, I think to myself.

One day later, as I'm pulling on my nightgown in preparation for bed, my arms feel like lead weights. I walk out of the bathroom and my legs throb. By morning, I ache everywhere—toes, fingers, teeth, eye-lids—and my hands and feet tingle. I feel as if I've been smashed beneath a five-ton steamroller.

The next day it's even worse. I take Motrin, eight hundred mil-ligrams every six hours, and hope it doesn't dissolve my stomach. It helps. At first. A little. After five interminable days the bone-crushing pain starts to recede.

The aches are successively worse after each Taxol infusion, and I end up taking Vicodan to sleep, even though I detest narcotics. The numbness in my hands and feet is worse, too. I drop spoons, can't knit on small needles, hit the wrong buttons on the computer keyboard. It feels as if I have no hands. I think of the teenager who, almost thirty years ago, was hitchhiking near Coalinga, California, near the school where my well-child clinic for migrant workers was held. She was picked up by a middle-aged man on a road I sometimes traveled. He got drunk, sexually assaulted her, and then took after her with an axe. She was found staggering along the edge of the highway with her arms cut off halfway between her wrists and elbows, blood dripping from the stumps.

I lie in bed rubbing my numb fingers and imagine what it would be like to actually have no hands. Those bleeding stumps loom in my mind. Such a horrid price to pay for a moment of bad decision making.

When I tell Ben about the numbness in my fingers, he wheels his stool next to me and asks me to undo one button of his shirt. This is a neuropathy test. Awkwardly, I push the button through its hole and then rebutton it again. A faint unease, a chill of caution, brushes over me. The maneuver is intimate and seems a little kinky, as if I'm undressing my doctor.

In the course of delivering medical care, physicians touch patients. Anywhere—even in the secret places. It's implicit in the covenant between doctors and the people they serve. The "laying on of hands" it's called, a very important component of the therapeutic process. Something magical flows through that skin-to-skin contact. To the patient, the physician's touch is soothing, affirming, reassuring, warm. Above all, it's safe, predicated on trust that the physician will not engage in inappropriate behavior, will act in the best interest of the patient, will respect professional boundaries.

Furthermore, the magic doesn't flow in only one direction. The examiner's touch also affects the physician. Besides relaying details of skin texture, muscle tone, and temperature, as well as clues to cardio-vascular, neurologic, and pulmonary function, that informative touch also reaffirms for the doctor that this is another human being, a person who depends on her, who trusts her as he may trust no other.

A patient, however, may *not* touch the doctor unless specifically asked to do so. A friendly, brief hug of appreciation is allowed. Touching the tip of the doctor's finger as it moves in front of the patient's face during coordination testing is also allowed, as is gripping a physician's fingers during strength testing. Unbuttoning one shirt button is allowed. Not much else.

Box elder bugs have invaded our home. On sunny days they flock to the south windows and poop on the glass. I pick one from my sleeve.

He jumps from my numb fingers and lands onto the table. His sienna-rimmed, brown shell swaggers as he crawls across the tabletop.

I'm about to get the vacuum cleaner, my favorite method for exterminating these insects. Then I see that he has only five limbs. Dragging his single right rear leg, he pulls himself toward my pencil holder with his four front feet. His progress is agonizingly slow, his gait tragically unsteady. What happened to his missing leg? He wasn't born that way, as such a severe disability would have kept him from getting into my house. How was his leg amputated? Probably by me. He might have been one of the many box elder bugs I have propelled across the room with a hearty flick of my finger. I decide not to exterminate this one. After limping to the edge of the table, he takes flight toward the sunny, south window.

The lady who faces me in the bathroom mirror, no hair and the left side of her bra half empty, stares out at me. I lean forward and carefully draw a brown line along the bare edges of my eyelids. I'm trying to make my eyes look more dramatic, less hairless. When finished, I lean back with my hands on my hips and survey my work. Then I notice my arms. They aren't the same size. In a T position, my arms extended from my sides, I internally and externally rotate my hands. I flex my elbows. My left arm definitely is bigger than my right.

I show Jim. He agrees that I have developed lymphedema. As a result of my axillary dissection, the damaged lymphatic channels that drain my left arm are clogged, so the lymph fluid backs up in my tissues.

I make an appointment with the occupational therapist to deal with this problem before I begin my radiation; the radiation burns to come will inflame my left upper chest, further impeding the lymph flow.

Rhonda measures the circumferences of both my arms; at ten centimeters above the elbow, my left upper arm is four centimeters bigger than my right. These values will be the baseline against which future measurements will be compared. She explains the therapeutic routine. Drink lots of water, limit caffeine-containing liquids. Don't lift heavy objects with the left arm. Don't carry a shoulder purse or computer case on the left side.

She massages my neck, clavicles, left armpit, left back, and left chest. She sets my left hand on her shoulder and slowly massages my arm, from axilla to fingertips and then in reverse. Her hands are soft, her strokes gentle and rhythmic as a rocking cradle. When she's finished, she cuts a thumbhole into a length of stockinette and pulls it on my arm. Then she wraps the arm in a four-inch-wide strip of foam and covers that with overlapping layers of Ace bandages. My arm, bulky and barely bendable, looks like a mummy.

This evening, one armed, I try to make meatloaf but have to use the mummified hand to steady the vegetables while I slice and dice. The palm wrappings will smell of onions for days, I suspect.

At my next visit, Rhonda strokes my arm again and explains, "We'll do the massages and the wraps three times a week until we see a nice decrease in the measurements of that arm and then we'll get you a compression sleeve."

"How long will I have to wear the compression sleeve?" I ask.

"Well . . . I would say for the duration."

"The duration? Of what? My life?"

"Well . . . yes."

# CHAPTER 15

*Friends, Forever*

*This month my book group* is reading *Disgrace* by the South African author J. M. Coetzee. I finished it yesterday evening and, even today, remain enraptured by its beauty. Yet, its story is dark and disturbing. Novels such as this upset me; it's the cleansing kind of upset that wrings one's marrow bloodless, only to be refilled by the liqueur of understanding. The powerful writing in this book, the horrific experiences of the characters, and their inability to comprehend each other reveal the deeply satisfying universal truths that lurk in good fiction.

Previously, the intensity of this book would have blown by me, ricocheting off my thoughts like rain off a slicker. I can't describe that former raincoat but recognize it by its absence, for without it, I'm exposed to all manner of watery encounters: mist, drizzle, cloud bursts, torrents, hail, tears.

Even the title word, *disgrace,* has grown more complex, because everything I meet is framed by my disease. Is having cancer a disgrace? Is having no hair a disgrace? Is being unable to accomplish my goals a disgrace? The answers to these questions languish in that murky zone between "yes" and "no."

The book group gathers at our house. Before we begin discussing *Disgrace,* Elizabeth announces she has a gift for me. She unfolds a sheet of paper on her lap and, in her rich, resonant voice, reads a poem that celebrates lying in bed. The words are lovely and aptly capture my new relationship with my mattress. As is true for the poet, for me my bed is a retreat; it's as secure as the inside of a womb; it's a place for time-out, for gathering wits; it's a recharging station for my body.

Other than marveling at the poem about the bed, the book group doesn't talk about my cancer. At our meetings everyone, including me, chooses to ignore the stinking, eight-hundred-pound gorilla that fills the living room of my life. My group offers me an escape from this terribly disordered reality and a return to the old, distantly familiar place where I'm normal and disease free, where I have a bright future, where I have hair. The fact is, however, that even though my cancer physically resides in the anatomic pathology laboratory at University Hospital, it's always with me, a gristled warp in my fabric, the engine that still drives most of my thoughts and actions.

My illness must be unsettling to the others in the group, as it rubs open the sore of their own vulnerabilities. If *I* could be hit so arbitrarily and unexpectedly with this disease, *they* could too. My bald head could be their bald head. My carved up chest could be their carved up chest. My courtship with death forces the realization that they, too, will die. One in the group was a mere teenager when her mother succumbed to breast cancer. Being with me must bring back difficult memories for her.

Sally and I attend a performance of the Czech Philharmonic Orchestra playing an all-Czech program. Afterward, her husband, Bill, and Jim join us for an afterglow in our kitchen. Bill uncorks a bottle of chardonnay. I spoon pepper and onion relish on a brick of cream cheese and spread a fan of crackers on a plate. We nibble and sip. And talk.

Sally and Bill have also endured cancer—three times, counting Bill's mother, who died when he was a boy. They understand what we're going through. We talk about the University Cancer Center, about our doctors and nurses, about the excellent care we have received there, about the snafus that occasionally clutter the way.

Jim opens a second bottle of chardonnay. We talk about our children. Their son and Daniel were buddies during elementary school and played on the same soccer and ice hockey teams. The boys' interests began to diverge during middle school, and they attended different high schools. While our sons were spending less and less time together, Bill and Sally and Jim and I grew closer. We camped together for a week in the Boundary Waters of northern Minnesota, canoeing and portaging by day, drinking wine from a box and wondering about moose by night. We skied for a week at Steamboat Springs, Colorado. Actually, they skied and I read, wrote, and knit, as I'm not a downhill skier and wasn't interested in starting at age fifty.

I open a bottle of Beaujolais, a jar of pickled onions, another sleeve of crackers, and a wedge of brie. We talk about growing up, me in Fargo, North Dakota; Jim in Valley City, North Dakota; Sally in Rochester, Minnesota; and Bill in West Virginia. We talk about our parents; Jim and Sally are the offspring of doctors, Bill of a dentist, and me of an x-ray equipment sales- and serviceman. We were all raised by stay-at-home mothers.

It's now four o'clock in the morning, and we have just finished tuna melt sandwiches, sliced apples, and a bottle of liebfraumilch. If Bill and Sally didn't live a half mile down the road, they would stay overnight, for we have all drunk too much. Alcohol doesn't make the cancer go away but, particularly in the company of dear friends, takes the sting out of it for a little while. Jim and I, more inebriated than we have been in decades, drop into our bed. We fall asleep, sated and content, my arm on his bare chest, his head against my shoulder.

My infectious diseases friend David calls me at home to ask how I'm doing. A woman in his laboratory had cancer several years ago, and he's very sensitive to the plight of someone undergoing chemotherapy. He tells me the interesting medical center gossip, the silly foibles of our leaders, the inexplicable antics of our colleagues; they strike me as very funny. I laugh so hard I can barely breathe. He speaks very fast, and I work like a plow horse to follow what he's saying. I don't want to miss a single word. When he says good-bye, I'm exhausted. The house is empty of sound. I head to bed for a nap.

Most of the other patients in the Cancer Center's infusion room are older than I, but Kathy is in her thirties. Her schedule is identical to mine, and she has occupied one of the Strato-Loungers during my most recent treatments. Today Kathy and her mother, who always accompanies her, are about seven or eight chairs down the line.

Kathy fascinates me. I envy her spunk. Today she wears a faded denim jumper, backless tennis shoes, and a floppy hat that sits crooked on her obviously bald head. She is clearly a favorite of the staff and jabbers continuously with her mother and the nurses, not bothering to lower her voice. Suddenly, she bursts into laughter and then, just as suddenly, sinks into solemnity. Her gaze fixes intently as a nurse explains something to her. Kathy nods. She reaches forward, her arm dotted with bruises the size of giant pansy blossoms, and takes the plastic cup of pills. She stares at the cup through narrowed eyes, shrugs, and calls out in her thundering voice, "Down the hatch." Then she dumps the pills into her mouth.

I treasure her honesty, the devil-may-care cock of her head, her glistening eyes, her inquisitive face, the easy swing of her body as she pushes her IV pole into the bathroom.

What kind of cancer does she have? She's young, vibrant, full of promise. Is there a man in her life? Why does she have to go through this? I yearn to know more about her, how she spends her time away from the Cancer Center, what she thinks about, what pleases her. But, Kathy remains a mystery to me, a bring-on-the-party woman who copes in her own lovely way with the terrible things that are happening to her.

When I leave for home, Kathy has wrapped a flannel blanket around her dainty, cancer-pocked body and sleeps while the poisons flow into her vein.

My chemotherapy infusion was only a week ago, but I'm on my way to Toronto to give my talk entitled "Periodic Fevers in Children." I was supposed to fly out of Detroit Metro last evening, but my flight, the last one of the day to Toronto, was canceled.

The lines at the Canadian Immigration Service in the Toronto airport are long and slow. Finally the officer in the booth calls me forward.

"Citizenship?" he asks.

"American."

"Passport, please."

Passport? Why should I need a passport? I have crossed the bridges from Michigan to Ontario many times and have never needed a passport.

"You need proof of citizenship to enter Canada," he says and points me to another line. Apparently the rules are different when you fly, as opposed to drive, into Canada.

By now I'm pooped. My afternoon nap is long overdue, and I haven't eaten all day for fear that airsickness will be additive to chemo sickness.

"Identification?" the next immigration officer asks. She is young and pretty in a well-scrubbed, homespun way.

I show her my Michigan driver's license, its photo taken when I still had eyebrows and hair. In my hat and chemo face, I look nothing like that picture.

"We need proof of citizenship," she says. "Anyone can get a U.S. driver's license, irrespective of their citizenship."

"I didn't realize I'd need my passport," I explain. "It's at home in Michigan." I'm embarrassed, as if I've done something hideously illegal and now have been caught. Eating humble pie is not something I'm good at.

"Why are you traveling to Canada?" She glances at my driver's license and doesn't seem to notice that I'm not the lady in the picture.

I explain that I'm attending ICAAC, the Inter-science Conference on Antimicrobial Agents and Chemotherapeutics. My legs ache. I'm woozy. I need to sit down.

"Can you prove that?" she asks.

I pull the ICAAC program book from my briefcase and show her my name. "I'm one of the speakers."

Her face brightens. "You're a doctor?"

"Yes."

"My cousin is a medical student at Dalhousie University."

This might be my ticket into this country. "I know several of the professors there." I take a deep breath. "In fact, the new dean of the medical school is a friend of mine."

"OK, doctor." She smiles. "Have a good time in Toronto and bring your passport on your next visit."


Trudy and I are staying in one of the downtown hotels. She arrived yesterday and stowed her things next to one of the beds. On the other bed she left a note:

> *Welcome to Toronto. Hope you got here safely.*
> *Is the inside bed OK with you?*
> *Love,*
> *Trudy*

I fold the note, climb under the quilt on the inside bed, and fall asleep.

Sometime later Trudy returns to the room. "Hi. You made it," she says as I sit up.

"I don't think I've registered for this meeting." I'm groggy from my nap. "I'd better do that or they won't let me into the lecture hall for my talk tomorrow. Where's the registration place?"

Trudy explains, and the more she talks, the deeper I sink into the cave of vulnerability. This is a huge meeting, with twelve thousand attendees. I'm not sure I can get over to the convention center and back by myself.

My face must show my confusion and frustration, because she stops talking and then says, "I'll go with you."

We walk four blocks through the afternoon crowds of downtown Toronto. It's noisy. The buildings reach for the sky; the setting sun is hidden behind their tall, concrete walls. Everyone is in a hurry. Buses and cars and taxis and trucks zoom past us in a blur.

"The convention center is through here," she says as we enter a building. I follow her along hallways, up escalators, along more hallways, around a corner, through a glassed-in atrium, and down escalators. For all I know, we're walking to Berlin.

"Here we are." We turn yet another corner and enter the registration area. She waits while I speak with the meeting officials. Turns out I, indeed, *have* registered for the meeting but didn't bring my book of abstracts or the badge card they said they sent to me.

This is so discouraging. I can't keep track of anything. I'm not sure if I received these materials in Ann Arbor or not.

Finally I finish the paperwork, and Trudy guides me back to our hotel. We arrive just in time for me to meet with the man, a former student, who is giving the other half of the talk on periodic fevers. He and I need to coordinate our presentations before tomorrow afternoon.

We review our slides and polish the lecture. When we're satisfied with the presentation, I offer him a Coke from the vending machine down the hall. Arun is one of my favorite people, smart, articulate, creative, and a genuinely nice man. When he laughs, his nutmeg-tinted face veers toward the ceiling, his ivory teeth gleam, and his dark, intense eyes disappear behind shuttered lids.

I explain what it's like to have cancer, to have every aspect of my life turned upside down, to be fatigued all the time, to be a stranger to my colleagues, to have no hair. He tells me of his family's inability to accept the one he loves. I buy another round of Cokes from the machine. It's dusk when he leaves and I'm exhausted. I order parsnip soup, a very Canadian dish, from room service. It's as creamy as the finest velvet ever made and tastes wonderful. Only faint grass clippings, only a little motor oil tint its flavor.

Trudy returns from her dinner meeting as I'm unpacking my suitcase: cosmetics bag in the bathroom, slacks and jackets on hangers in the closet, underwear in the dresser drawer, night gown on the bed.

"Damn it, Trudy, I forgot to bring my night hat."

"Your what?"

"The knit bonnet I wear to bed."

"Janet," she says kindly, "if you're comfortable with your head uncovered, it's fine with me."

I pause. No one except Jim has seen me bald. I watch Trudy as she sits on the bed. Her back is propped against the pillows, her ankles are crossed, the meeting book rests in her lap, and a sweet smile warms her face. We've been friends for over twenty years and always stay together at infectious diseases meetings. During a particularly difficult time, she and I spent a week at Lake Five, Minnesota, a hundred acres of water and only ten cabins. Loons were all over the place, and there were no motorboats, no televisions or phones, and no locks on the doors. For six days we knitted scarves and cooked wild rice and hiked and picked wood ticks off our arms and canoed and tried to straighten out tangled lives.

I look at her again, at her accepting grin, at the easy set of her shoulders. Why should I hesitate showing her my head? She's one of my best friends, someone who has revealed many secrets to me. We're both physicians, have taken care of people with disfiguring scars, with missing ears and noses and limbs, with ghastly burns, with cruel infections, and we have not made judgments about them.

I pull off my straw hat, the one with maroon peonies pinned to the brim, and send it sailing to the bed. Then I yank off my rose print scarf, unmasking my baldness.

Trudy lays down her book. The vain part of me wants to run for cover; the secure part wants to stand proud.

She smiles again. "You have a lovely head. A really, really beautiful head."

Together we laugh.

The next afternoon I don my wig and one of my new pantsuits. Trudy guides me once again to the convention center and deposits me at the lecture hall where I'm to give my talk. Arun is already there and helps me load my PowerPoint disk.

The room fills with people, and those without seats line the walls. Two of our trainees from Michigan are in the second row. Like Tweedle-Dee and Tweedle-Dum, they each give me a silly wave.

I begin with a few introductory remarks and then launch into my talk. Standing there at the podium, a microphone before me and a laser pointer in my hand, I'm suddenly transformed back to the real me. It's as if the awful months since last Valentine's Day never happened, as if they were spliced from my life. I'm confident. I'm talking about a subject I know well. I'm a pediatric infectious diseases doctor again, an academic physician, an educator. The right words come to me effortlessly. I click through my slides, emphasizing the important points, repeating the *really* important points. By the time I reach the conclusions, I'm radiant.

Arun walks me back to my hotel. Overhead, wispy clouds race between the tall buildings, pushed by an Ontario gale. I turn away from the wind so it blows against the back of my head and then turn again when the wind shifts. I'm worried my wig will be blown away. At the crosswalk, we stop for a red light and an up-current whips around the corner. I plop my hand on the top of my head. My wig is secured against the squall, and the light turns green. We cross the street.

The next morning I return to the Toronto airport on the shuttle bus. We pass a domed football stadium and billboards advertising Molsen beer. Like most Canadian cities, Toronto is clean. True to that country's quirky character, men tell jokes and punch each other in the shoulder. Well-dressed women wear clothes that are about fifteen degrees off from today's American fashions, sometimes more frilly, sometimes more finely cut. They talk like Americans, only different. They walk like Americans, only different. Toronto is foreign, but the degree of its foreignness sits midscale between the two opposing worlds I juggle at home—the new one filled with cancer and the old one I left behind.

Cars line the passenger pick-up lane at Detroit Metro airport, but Jim's van isn't among them. On the sidewalk, between the thick, concrete columns, one bench is empty; the others are occupied by people drawing cigarette smoke into their lungs and blowing it out into the auto exhaust and jet fuel polluted air. I take a seat on the empty bench and begin to knit while I wait for Jim.

A man pulls his suitcase to a stop beside me, sits down on my bench, and lights up a cigarette.

Should I say something to him? This may be a public place, but, in my view, he is being thoughtless to start smoking where there are no smokers. In many situations I'm not highly assertive, as I've learned to put up with a lot of marginal behavior. Still . . . this irritates me.

Finally, I can't stand it any longer.

"Sir," I say.

He flicks his ash on the sidewalk and turns toward me.

I take a deep breath. "I'm being treated for one type of cancer and have no interest in getting another one, ever. There's plenty of room on the other benches where people are smoking."

He turns the color of raspberries, apologizes, and moves to the next bench.

I haven't seen my friend Eleanor for about a year; when she hears about my cancer, she takes me to lunch. I explain that, since my surgery, my nipples now point in different directions. "Looks as if my headlights are sprung."

"So do mine," she laughs. "Always have."

At the end of my clinic appointment I report to the Cancer Center reception desk. The clerk takes my checkout papers and continues talking on the phone—something about trouble with one of her sisters. She stares at the computer monitor, types a few keystrokes, stares again, and keeps talking into the phone. Finally she passes me a paper with information about my next appointment. During this entire three-minute encounter, she hasn't made eye contact with me, has not spoken to me. Why does this have to happen? And why does it happen here, where I work? It infuriates me to be treated this way; worse, my patients are probably treated this way.

It's no different here than at other medical centers, as the health-care system everywhere in America is badly dysfunctional. The explanation is simple. When you try to provide increasingly expensive care to more and sicker people, but with fewer resources, the implosion is resounding.

This move to Wal-Mart medicine saddens me and all my physician colleagues, for it clashes with our traditions of altruistic medical practice. It's not consistent with the way we learned to be doctors.

✿

"I'm coming to visit you," Kay says. She's calling from her home near Dallas, Texas. "Tell me when."

Kay is married to the obstetrician who delivered Daniel at Mountain Home Air Force Base in Idaho. After our son's birth, John and Kay and their toddler daughter accepted our invitation for a weekend of fishing on the Indian reservation where we lived in Nevada. From then until we moved to Alaska eighteen months later, they spent at least one weekend every month with us. We have been friends for twenty-five years. It's the kind of friendship that requires only semiannual phone calls to stay firmly glued together.

"You know, Kay, a good time would be while Jim's in Montana with his brothers." I'm thrilled that she will visit. "Jim's hesitant about leaving. While he's away he'll feel more comfortable if you're here with me."

"What should we do while I'm in Michigan? Are you up for a trip?" she asks. "I'm game for whatever you want."

"There's one thing I would love to do." I'm equally thrilled that Kay is so flexible; I'm confident she will indulge one of my passions, something few other people would be willing to endure. "Let's spend a couple days at Sault Ste. Marie, watching the lakers go through the locks."

"Sounds fun," Kay says, even though undoubtedly she doesn't know what lakers are.

Several days before Kay arrives, Jim and I join Daniel at the San Jose, California, airport and drive to Monterey for Joe's graduation from the Defense Language Institute. It's been only five days since my chemo infusion, and I ache everywhere. But nothing—not wild horses, not chemotherapy—could keep me from being here. As we leave the airport, I curl up in the backseat of our rental car, my purse for a pillow.

About halfway to the Monterey Peninsula I smell garlic. "Hey," I call into the front seat. "We must be in Gilroy."

"Yessiree," Daniel calls over his shoulder from the driver's seat.

I have reserved a room for Jim and me at a swanky bed and breakfast. Jim agrees that I have earned a couple of days surrounded by luxury. Daniel has a room at a Day's Inn down the road. I spend much of the weekend buried in the downy bed but manage to get up for the graduation ceremony.

The Presidio of Monterey's auditorium, known as the Tin Barn, is standard, down-at-the-heels military decor. We arrive early and take our seats on the folding chairs. As the other families file in, I remember the old joke about sitting in a movie theater behind the fat lady with the hat. I'm wearing my white straw hat with the huge organdy, midnight blue bow and worry about the people behind me; they want to see their son or daughter stroll across the stage as much as I want to see Joe. Should I take the hat off and sit in my scarf? I don't want to embarrass Joe; on his special day I want him to have a normal mom. So I watch the ceremony while standing against the government-green cinderblock wall where I obstruct no one's view.

The flight home from California is complicated. Almost simultaneously, Dan takes off from San Jose to fly to Portland, Oregon; Jim leaves for Montana; and I leave for Detroit. My dose of G-CSF comes due during my layover in Minneapolis, so I sit on the toilet in an airport stall, my Rollaboard shoved against the door, my purse and knitting bag hung on the hook, and give myself the shot. Where should I put the empty syringe? Not in the trash here. Not down the drain. This public bathroom isn't equipped for the realities of modern medicine in which patients receive treatment at unexpected places. So I stow it in my purse until I can deposit it at home in the empty orange juice bottle where I keep the others.

While waiting in the boarding area, I scrutinize the other passengers. There are hundreds of them, rushing here, rushing there, waiting in line, chatting on cell phones. They are short, tall, fat, thin, beautiful, and homely, but none have the telltale signs of chemotherapy. Surely at least a few have cancer, ovarian or prostate, colon or lung, but it doesn't show.

As the plane jets eastward over Lake Michigan, I'm giddy with anticipation. It's been at least a decade since Kay and I were last together, ten years of change. Our waists will both be thicker, our jowls will have sagged, her hair will be streaked with gray—mine is gone. She'll be good company during the long empty days while Jim is away, and her old ankle injury will keep us at the same pace—SLOW. She has arranged to arrive into Detroit Metro about an hour before me and will meet me at my gate.

After my plane stops at the terminal, I set my hat, which has rested on my knees during the flight, back on my head, pull my suitcase from the overhead compartment, walk down the aisle, trot up the jetway, and, breathless with expectation, burst into the boarding area.

No Kay. Where is she? I wait for half an hour and then walk, hauling my suitcase and knitting bag, to the American Airlines gates to see if her plane has been delayed. It hasn't. I ask the agent if she was on the plane, fully expecting that he'd refuse to give me that information. Instead, he looks at me, at the gaunt, sunken-eyed, scarved-and-hatted woman before him and begins typing at his computer. Yes, he tells me, she was on her scheduled flight. So where is she now?

I haul my Rollaboard down to the American Airlines luggage claim area. No Kay. I call the airport paging system to make an overhead announcement. Still no Kay. Finally, exhausted, frustrated, puzzled, worried, and out of ideas about where to find her, I drive home.

Ten minutes after arriving at my house, the phone rings.

"Hi," says Kay. "Glad you made it home."

"Where *are* you?"

"In the lobby of your hospital."

I stutter, "The hospital . . . Why are you there?"

"Well . . . ," she says in her key lime pie, Florida drawl, "I forgot to bring your flight information so I had no idea which plane you were on and I couldn't remember which airport you were flying in from."

"From San Jose with a connection in Minneapolis."

"Oh . . . right. I thought it was somewhere in California, so I checked all the San Francisco and Los Angeles flights and you weren't on them. I took the shuttle from the airport to your hospital. I also forgot to bring your home phone number, so I sweet-talked the reception-ist into giving it to me."

"Kay, FYI for the next time, it's in the Ann Arbor phone book." Now that my worry has dissolved, I can't be upset with her. Kay is Kay.

"How do I get to your house?" she asks. "Tell me the address and I'll take a cab."

"No way. Stay put. I'll pick you up in ten minutes."

I pull my car into the medical center's circle drive. There she stands, framed by the hospital's entrance, dressed in pink, her suitcase at her feet. I race into her open arms, and her head knocks against my hat, jostling it to the ground.


After several days of talking and knitting and eating her terrific food, Kay and I load Jim's van for the trip to Sault Ste. Marie. We can't take my car because it has a standard transmission, thus requiring one of the few life skills Kay has failed to master.

Three hours into the six-hour trip, we pull off the highway, head-ing toward a rest stop. The road curves upward through the pines and ends in the parking lot at the top of a hill. A hawk glides along the tree-tops, banking to the left, turning, then banking to the right. Off in the distance, beyond the stripe of freeway far below, the sun's rays bounce off the surface of a lake buried in the woods. The breeze that carries the hawk wafts against our cheeks. Kay loves being away from sweltering Dallas in July and marvels at the clear, crisp Michigan-in-summer air.

"Can I stay here forever?"

"Fine with me," I answer. "You might want to discuss it with your husband."


A bit farther down the road the "check engine" light blinks on.

"What's that all about?" Kay asks.

"No idea."

I rummage through Jim's glove compartment for the owner's manual. Not there.

She takes the next freeway exit and pulls into a gas station. Ignorant of car engines, Kay and I stand elbow to elbow in front of the open hood and stare into the innards of Jim's van.

"Maybe we should check the oil," I suggest.

The dipstick shows that the oil level is very low, so we buy two bottles of Pennzoil and fill 'er up. I store this incident in my mental "take it up with Jim later" file. He will have some apologizing to do.

The "check engine" light stays off the remainder of the trip, and we arrive in Sault Ste. Marie late in the afternoon.

Our bed and breakfast, a turn-of-the-century mansion with a huge stained glass window in the main stairwell, is across the street from the St. Mary's River. We could sit on the front porch and watch the freighters approach the locks, but it isn't close enough for me. Instead, we settle on a park bench four feet from the water's edge and wait and knit. As our fingers loop the yarn over the needles, we talk about our kids, our husbands, our fish dinners back in Nevada, their escape-prone English setter that we chased for miles across the Grand Forks Air Force Base, the foggy mornings at their house in the shadow of the Golden Gate Bridge. Stitch by stitch, row by row, our pieces grow.

The first up-bound ship to go through the locks is the *Oglebay Norton*, a thousand-foot "laker," longer than three football fields. Its raisin-colored hull rounds the bend in the river headed for the Poe Lock. Its bow parts the water effortlessly, silently. This freighter, like all the others, is utterly majestic—massive, soundless, insistent, proud. Its radar antenna twirls above the pilothouse, sampling the air like a snake's tongue. The net of a basketball hoop mounted on the tower's wall sways in the wind, ready to absorb the crew's boredom as soon as they are under way again. On the deck, the seamen lean lazily against the rail and the pilot sits at the controls, his elbow resting on the open windowsill. Kay and I wave like excited three-year-olds. The crew members smile and wave back.

The next afternoon we explore the Soo Locks Visitors Center. Standing on the viewing platform, we stare down on the deck of the

*Agawa Canyon* below, in the MacArthur Lock. Slowly, slowly, the ship, trapped between the gates of the lock, is lifted by the rising water from the level of Lake Huron to that of Lake Superior, twenty-one feet higher.

After a nap, we tour an old laker that has been made into a museum. Peeking into the restored crew quarters, I imagine my Uncle John, a sailor in the merchant marines, sleeping on one of the cots or eating from the metal plates at the mess table. There is his heavy, rubber coat hanging from a hook. There are his boots, shoved under the bed. I was in love with Uncle John as a young girl. He's the one who, serious as an undertaker, read books to Nancy and me backwards while we shrieked with glee. He's the one who taught us to spell Mississippi—M-I-crooked letter-crooked letter-I-crooked letter-crooked letter-I-humpback-humpback-I. My favorite place in Grandma Reed's house was his old bedroom, where his navy cap and World War II medals were displayed on the dresser. He died in his forties—a broken man, his liver battered from alcohol—at least ten years after I last saw him. I'm sure he's the reason I'm so drawn to the lakers.

In the morning, before the maids come, Kay and I prowl through the mansion where we are staying. We snoop into unoccupied rooms and follow back staircases. Later we drive to the Point Iroquois Lighthouse on Lake Superior and peer into the light keeper's quarters. The kitchen, with its spice cans, Fel's naphtha soap, wringer washing machine, metal breadbox, and console radio as big as a suitcase, is the twin of my mother's kitchen when I was a child.

"Want to go up?" I ask as we near the stairs to the light tower.

"No," Kay says. "Do you?"

"Nope." Neither of us is in condition for the climb, and at this point in our lives we don't need to scale lofty heights to prove anything to anyone. Rather, we're content to stand on the ground and admire from below the light beam as it pulses out over the shoals of Lake Superior.

On the way back to Sault Ste. Marie, Kay insists on stopping at a fenced-in area on the Bay Mills Reservation. The faded sign says "Old Indian Cemetery." The gate is open so we walk into the cool, dark grove of evergreens and maple trees on the Lake Superior shore. The fish-tainted squalls off the water blow through the pines and send skittering the dried leaves that litter the ground. At our feet rest ancient gravestones and short wooden houses the size of baby coffins.

"Do you know what these are for?" Kay whispers, echoing the reverence that a cemetery demands.

"No," I whisper back. "Must be burial boxes or something."

Kay gets down on her hands and knees and peers into the hole on the side of one of the boxes. I don't want to look.

"What's in there?" I whisper.

"Can't tell," she whispers back. "Too dark."

On the way back to Ann Arbor, I become sullen. I don't want to go home. I want to stay "up north" where the lakers ride the now smooth water that used to be the St. Mary's rapids. I want to stay where there is no chemo, no Cancer Center, no waiting rooms, no examining rooms; where having no hair doesn't bother me at all; where, except for fatigue and G-CSF injections, I can feel normal.

As Jim's van barrels south on I-75, I look over at Kay, her hands gripping the steering wheel, her eyes staring straight ahead through the windshield. She is talking about her granddaughter, the child of the red-headed little girl who came fishing on the reservation in Nevada so many, many years ago. Kay is laughing.

⚘

Alice slaps the back of my right hand, trying to raise her favorite vein. She locates it, slips in the IV needle, and the Taxol starts to flow. As she works, she speaks of her daughter.

"I got a call from the sheriff yesterday. She's in the county jail again."

I lean back in the Strato-Lounger.

"She can't seem to get away from those awful friends of hers. The dealers and users."

I rub my nose.

"I'm such a bad mother," she says.

I shift to the other hip.

"She calls me at work. Upsets me so much I can barely get through the day."

I straighten my scarf.

"Should I bail her out again?" Alice asks, although she doesn't expect an answer from me.

Jim doesn't accompany me to my infusions anymore. Friday afternoon is his clinic, and I don't want him to cancel every third clinic to be with me. Driving home alone isn't an issue because I don't get sick immediately after the drugs are infused.

Valerie, a fellow faculty member in pediatrics, sits in the chair at the foot of my Strato-Lounger and fills me in on the news from the department. Her clinic is just around the corner from the infusion room, and she has stopped by to spend a little time with me. Others have sat here during my infusions as well: Kay while she visited, Larry from Peds Hem-Onc, Nan from my book group who is also a university physician.

After Valerie leaves, I think again of Natalie, the pediatrician from Fresno who died of cancer. Her story, or at least a distorted version of her story, is the source of my cancer illusion, the one in which I'm driving home from a chemo treatment, by myself with the vomit pail in my lap. Since I first read about Natalie I have anticipated that, for me, chemotherapy would mean being sick and alone, whereas she had a gaggle of friends who supported her through it.

I cling to this illusion as a burr sticks to wool. The evidence is abundant that I have many friends who have been wonderful to me in myriad creative, thoughtful ways. And yet. And yet. That old illusion seems to be acid-etched deep inside me. I can't make it go completely away. It will always be there.

This is my last chemo infusion. It's the last time I have to wait in the Cancer Center reception area among the other patients—the anemic, the gray, the yellow, the bald; the last time to sit in the Strato-Lounger with poisons dripping into my vein. Alice gives me a farewell hug, and I wish her well with her daughter.

This is an ending, and like most people—novelists, lovers, travelers, relatives of the terminally ill, parents of children going off to college—I don't handle endings well. The end of anything means the beginning of something else, and for some of us, change is difficult; we prefer the familiar walls that line the ruts of our lives. Inherent in an ending is the disappointment that the road getting there wasn't perfect and that its flaws can never be redressed. I have always dealt with endings by ignoring them. When I leave—a party, a school, a relationship, a town—I dispense with good-byes and just disappear.

On Sunday after my last dose of chemo, as the drug effects are beginning to cramp my muscles and numb my hands and feet, my writing group suggests we all go out to dinner the next time we meet, to "celebrate" the end of my chemotherapy. I nod and change the subject. Hopefully this thought will die the natural death of an unwanted idea.

I don't want to celebrate. In completing my chemotherapy, I haven't done anything great; I've barely tolerated getting through it. The writing group longs to do something nice for me, but I can't begin to describe to them how uncelebratory I feel. I just want to move on, to slog forward to the next step in therapy. It is, after all, one of those endings—badly done.

# CHAPTER 16

❧

## *And Then They Burn You*

*The chemotherapy phase of my treatment* is over, and I'm ready for the radiotherapy phase. I hand my clinic checkout papers to the clerk in the Cancer Center. "I need an appointment with Dr. Edwards in radiation oncology."

The tap of the clerk's fingernails on the computer keyboard melts into the surrounding din. The typing stops . . . then starts again . . . then stops.

"Dr. Edwards isn't available," she says. "She's on maternity leave for several months. Dr. Stenholm is available."

What? This makes no sense. During my appointment with Jackie, six months ago when I was first diagnosed with cancer, we agreed she would be my radiation oncologist. She gave no indication she would be off work for a while.

The clerk keeps typing. "Shall I set it up with Dr. Stenholm?"

I'm stunned, thrown completely off-kilter. How can this be? "I guess so," I stammer.

Did I get something mixed up? Jackie has a young child, and it's certainly possible she would expand her family. Maybe at my first appointment she didn't know she was pregnant. Maybe she's had a difficult pregnancy and needed to stop working suddenly and earlier than expected.

The clerk hands me the information for my appointment with Dr. Stenholm.

Three weeks later, Jim sits beside me in the radiation oncology examining room. Shuffling through my records, Dr. Stenholm says, "I see that you had an appointment previously with Dr. Edwards."

"Yes," I say. "I understand she's away on maternity leave for several months."

"No, she's not," he says quickly. "She's in Europe . . . at a cancer investigators' meeting. She'll be back next week."

I feel like an idiot. An enraged idiot. I thought I knew all the land mines in the medical system here, thought that if I kept my head up I would see them coming and step aside. That clerk was very confident when she gave me the wrong information about my doctor, her fingernails clicking on the keyboard all the while. How could I predict such a blunder? Should I believe *nothing* I'm told? Do I, as the patient, need to triple-check everything?

The next week, probably seconds after returning from her trip, Jackie sends me an e-mail asking about the appointment with Dr. Stenholm. I call her and explain the unbelievable situation. The anger in her voice rattles the phone circuitry, but she remains diplomatic. "I'll set you up for an appointment with me right away."

The first stage in radiation therapy is the "simulation," during which measurements are taken to develop a treatment plan. At this appointment I'm shoved into the donut hole of the CT scanner, my first personal experience with this machine. There isn't a lot of room inside. Fortunately it wraps around my chest so that my head sticks out the top end. Otherwise I would fall victim to claustrophobia. As the equipment churns and sputters around me, I try to attach interesting images to the sounds, to visualize the waves of the Pacific Ocean that lap against the sailboats moored at Moss Landing, that ripple over the sandy beach in Monterey, that crash into the rocks at Point Lobos.

Today's CT scan will be used to design my treatments, to calculate the exact paths the radiation beams must take to attack any leftover cancer and yet avoid normal tissues. Since full-force radiation could be very destructive to my heart, my lungs, and the bone marrow in my ribs, the rays will enter my body at different angles and focus on the place where the tumor used to be. It's reminiscent of the way my childhood friend Mary Euren and I, as eight-year-olds on her driveway, murdered ants by zapping them with sunbeams converged through a magnifying glass.

During this appointment, my "cradle," a sponge form in which I will lie during my treatments, is cast. The technicians align me in the casting mold, my right arm at my side and my left arm bent upward in a scratching-the-top-of-your-head position. They nudge my arm here, push my chest there, as I lie motionless. A sheet of plastic wrap separates me from the goo that will become my cradle. The goo begins to stir—a chemical reaction has begun. It's barely perceptible at first, and then the goo slowly heats up, warming my skin like bathwater. Ultimately, the sticky foam stiffens into a bowl that cups my back and the sides of my chest and forms a trough for my bent left arm.

Jackie glides into the darkened room. Her presence—commanding, efficient, calm—reassures me as she instructs the technicians about the measurements. Then, using a Sharpie pen, she swiftly, deftly draws the blue lines on my chest that will define the radiation field.

My next appointment is for "verification," the process of confirming the planned tracks of the radiation beams. The technician pulls my cradle from its slot along the wall, from a row of molds, one for each patient currently receiving radiation therapy, and slams it on the table. I climb into my form and am told not to move *at all*, as they will be taking many x-rays and even the slightest motion will make the films impossible to read. This will last about an hour, they say, which I suspect is a low estimate, as the truth would be too discouraging.

After twenty minutes, my neck is sore as hell. In an attempt at distraction, I sneak a deep breath when they aren't actually snapping a film. That doesn't help. Then I imagine—but don't actually do it—moving my head. That doesn't help, either. I can't stand this. I'll never be able to last the hour. I wiggle my big toes a tiny, tiny bit; surely my feet are far enough away from my chest that a slight motion at the ends of my legs won't skew the alignment. The pain continues to drill at the base of my skull.

I try visualization again, imagining what my head looks like in the mold, hoping these thoughts will pass the time and make the pain endurable. That also doesn't help, but as I'm imagining my bald skull in the goo while it solidified several days ago, I realize that today, as opposed to earlier, I'm wearing a head scarf, and its knot sits exactly at the sore spot in my neck.

During a lull in the film taking, I say to the technician, "I'm not going to be able to stand this any longer. Could you remove my scarf? The knot is driving me nuts."

Her fingers are warm and nimble as they pull the scarf, and the knot, away from my scalp without moving me. My bald head settles into the foam, and the pain disappears. Such a tiny gesture; such a huge relief.

After what seems like a thousand x-ray shots and two hours, I'm allowed to sit up from the cradle for a short while.

Next come the tattoos. These marks will guide the technicians in correctly positioning the angle of the radiation beams during my treatments. The technician is sweet and funny as she dabs three drops of India ink on my skin and jabs the point of an eighteen-gauge needle into each drop. Often, when people learn that Daniel, our son who has many elaborate images inked on his skin, is a tattoo artist, they ask if I have one. Now I can truthfully answer, "Yes, I have several." When they ask what my tattoos look like, I will say, "Three fleas."

"Good news," Jackie says after reviewing the verification films and adjusting the blocks of lead that will shield the vulnerable organs of my chest from the beam. "We are able to include that medial lymph node in the treatment field without delivering too much radiation to your heart." She's referring to the extra pinto bean that appeared beside my sternum during the sentinel node scan many months ago. Maybe now I can stop worrying about it.

The treatments themselves are simple. I climb into the cradle, watch the technician position the eye of the linear accelerator, hold my breath, listen to the whir of the machine, breathe again. She repositions the beam and I repeat the breathing routine. She repositions the beam again and I repeat the breathing routine for the third time. Then I climb out of the cradle.

The radiation oncology technicians remind me of the Jawas, those funny little creatures in the *Star Wars* movie who dart around in brown robes and whose shiny eyes flash from deep inside their hoods. The technicians scurry out of the darkened room before "the beam" of the linear accelerator comes on and then scurry back in to reposition the machine. Their whispery voices echo through the room, and I hear only fragments of what they say. I lie in my cradle, motionless, and sense their flitting movements at the edges of my vision.

❧

In my journal I write:

*HALLOWEEN.*
*I could go trick-or-treating as a breast cancer patient . . .*
- *No hair*
- *No eyebrows*
- *No eyelashes*
- *Blue Sharpie lines drawn all over my scarred chest*
- *Faded, threadbare hospital gown gaping open in front between the ties.*

❧

Even more than the chemotherapy waiting room, I dislike the radiation oncology waiting room. The fact that it's run very efficiently and staffed by friendly people doesn't dispel my dislike. The Scotch-guarded floral upholstery, the composite-wood-with-oak-veneer tables, and the Holiday Inn–like pastel pictures on the wall—pseudo chic with forced elegance—irritate me. In my hospital gowns, the inner one on backward, the outer one on frontward as a flimsy concession to modesty, I sit among other patients and their families who compare cancer stories as they wait. Huddled in the corner behind my book, I pretend to read.

One woman waits for her daughter who traveled from Puerto Rico to Ann Arbor for her treatment. She describes the abysmal medical care she received at home. Another tells of her daughter-in-law whose breast cancer progressed to new neck nodes while on chemotherapy. She describes the weeping burns on her daughter-in-law's chest, her own husband's death from cancer, her son's death at age twenty-one from cancer.

Is this a "who suffers most" contest? If so, it's a game I have no interest in playing. All of them can win, as far as I'm concerned. They're talking about the one thing we have in common, and I opt out. Where can I go to get away from these stories, from these patients? A stall in the bathroom? One of the curtained cubicles in the dressing room? No. I have to stay here so I can hear my name being called.

The daughter-in-law, one-inch fuzz sprouting on her head, returns to the waiting room after her treatment. With one hand, she holds her hospital gown away from her blistered chest; with the other, she digs for her pain pills in the bottom of her purse. She's going to die of her breast cancer; in the end, it will prevail. Yet she keeps fighting it, keeps subjecting herself to the burning.

To hide is to keep a secret, to try to maintain dignity. In my journal I make a list.

*Things I can hide:*
- *Chemo brain: the lost words, the missing names, the facts and concepts—once learned, now forgotten*
- *The scars—on my chest, in my armpit, throughout my being*
- *Stinging hurts that come, like stealth missiles, from unexpected people and places*
- *Numb, fumbling fingers*
- *Chemo ridges in toenails*
- *The little things in need of repair: broken zippers, holes in socks, torn panty elastic, fallen hems that are secured with Scotch tape*

*Things I can't hide:*
- *No eyelashes*
- *No eyebrows*
- *The weary, hollow-eyed stare of a bald cancer patient*

It's been nine endless months since I was diagnosed with cancer, and I'm still undergoing treatment, a seemingly infinite exercise in endurance. Five days a week I report to the radiation oncology department, check in at the desk, change into a hospital gown and hang my clothes in a locker, sit in the horrible waiting room, spend fifteen minutes lying in my cradle under the linear accelerator while the beams race through my chest, change back into my clothes, and then go home to rest.

The skin on my chest is sore from the radiation, and I can no longer tolerate my bra. I'm back to wearing tank-top undershirts, the ribbed knit, scooped neck kind my Grandpa Reed used to wear. I dab aloe gel on my sore breast as instructed. I'm not convinced it does any good, other than cooling my fiery skin, but I use it anyway.

My radiation therapy appointments are usually after lunch so that patients who come from farther away can be treated early and be on the road to home before noon. Occasionally the technicians call to reschedule my time because they know I'm in my office before my treatments and easy to track down. I don't mind changing my schedule for the sake of the other patients; it's easy for me to do, and I feel noble in doing them a favor. I just don't like sitting in the waiting room while they chatter. When I'm the doctor, I love hearing my patients' stories. That's how I learn who they are; it's how I figure out the most effective way to help them with their medical problems. When I'm the patient in the chair next to them in the waiting room, however, I don't want to listen to their tales.

Across the street, our neighbor's lawn mower sits abandoned in his yard. Grass four inches tall sways ahead of it; a neat, mowed swath lies behind. Overhead, a flock of geese, arrayed in a sloppy V, heads south.

At the rear of the V, a lone straggler flaps his wings for all he's worth, trying to catch up with the rest. Why is he straggling? Is he weak? Or sick? Or did he get a late start?

"My cancer doesn't define me," I tell my oncologist. "It's not who I am."

He nods.

"It's a bit of a complication in my life, but not a keynote event."

He nods again.

"So, you won't see me marching in cancer survivor parades."

He smiles and nods.

"Besides that, I find the term *cancer survivor* distasteful. It suggests I did something terrific to still be alive. I did no such thing. I merely followed your instructions."

He nods.

"And what about those poor souls who are *cancer deaths*? Are they diminished as people, weak or incompetent or misdirected or of no value, because they didn't survive?"

He nods yet again. As my doctor, he respects whatever I say, just as he respects the decisions of the women who march in the pink-ribbon parades.

Before he leaves the examining room, he gives me a hug. It's a lovely expression of caring; of admiration for me who has gone through hell, by him who directed some of that hell; of his respect for me in the face of my childlike dependency on him.

Beyond the radiation oncology waiting room, the doctors, my medical colleagues, dart in and out of doorways, give orders, make decisions, are important. They wear clinician uniforms, long white coats. I wear my hospital gown. I want to be one of them again, making diagnoses, interpreting laboratory tests, taking medical histories, performing physical examinations, devising treatment plans. Instead, I wait.

Waiting. Life at a standstill. It's the same as being mired crotch-deep in quicksand until someone comes to pull you out. It's enduring gridlock on a crowded freeway at rush hour. It's languishing in line at the secretary of state's office to replace a lost driver's license. It's what you do while receiving cancer therapy.

As we wait, the people in this holding tank of a room, including me, are slaves to the schedules and needs and agendas of others. Furthermore, we are undressed. At University Hospital, I'm accustomed to being fully clothed and to having patients wait for *me*. There is absolutely no dignity here. I'm not in control. I'm left out. I don't belong.

※

"Walk," my oncologist told me when my treatment began. "I want you to walk. We know that cancer patients do better when they are physically active."

So I walk. Sometimes I hike the trails in the university's botanical gardens. Sometimes I trek the entire loop through Gallup Park. Today I'm walking in Parker Mill Park.

I pass the old cider mill and the older grist mill; "1887" and "1873" are inscribed on their cornerstones. I wander past the log cabin at the edge of the now vacant picnic area. At the fork in the path, I turn left onto the Hoyt G. Post trail, a wooden boardwalk that follows Fleming Creek for a while before it heads deep into the woods. Fallen leaves, crisp, still, colored many shades of tan, blanket the understory like discarded scabs.

I stop at the platform that juts over a turn in the creek and watch the water swirl among the rocks and tree stumps. I pass the apple orchard that once stood beside the long-gone mill pond and fed the cider presses. Last spring, pink blossoms, barely visible above the bushes, dotted the tree branches. Now the branches, cracked and gnarled, are bare.

Inside the quarry rock cavern, with the Amtrak rail bed overhead, the air is heavy, damp, and cool. Beside me, Fleming Creek gurgles past the stone pylons as it rushes, restlessly, relentlessly, toward the Huron River. Except for the droning low of the creek, it's quiet. Beyond the path to the old wooden duck blind, the boardwalk takes a bend. As I round the corner, I surprise three deer grazing on the wild ginger. They bounce through the woods toward the other side of the park, their hooves clattering on the planks of the walkway. They leave with their tails up, the white patches that slash down their tawny buttocks waving good-bye.

❧

I'm very tired of my hats. They are lovely and elicit many compliments from friends and from strangers, but they make me feel odd. Normal people don't wear hats like these, especially to concerts, to dinner at nice restaurants, to the bookstore, to the veterinarian's office, to T. J. Maxx. Appearing different from most people isn't what bothers me—after all, I *like* distinction, of the positive kind. Rather, the hats give me the air of a social misfit, a person with an attitude trying to draw attention to herself, a woman making an outlandish visual statement.

On the other hand, I kind of enjoy wearing my hats in airports. It's a deviant, twisted kind of enjoyment. When I board a plane, I consider my hat to be a badge of honor. Its presence on my scarved head is like shouting to the strangers around me, "I have cancer. I have no hair. And, yet, I have a life and will travel."

❧

I've been stuck in this examining room for thirty minutes and am getting edgy. Outside the door, a gaggle of Cancer Center employees chatter and laugh. Impatient, I open the door and say, "It's been half an hour. Hopefully I've not been forgotten." In my clinic we sometimes joke about fictional patients being stranded for a month behind the closed door of an examining room. It's the clinic version of "falling through the cracks." Today the joke isn't funny.

"Oh, no, we haven't forgotten," one of the medical assistants says. "Dr. Miller is running late today."

Now it's been an hour. I'm not idly staring at the wall, of course, but have read the morning's *New York Times* and three medical papers and am now working on my knitting. I've learned to come prepared for a wait, but this is excessive. The employees are still outside my room, still complaining about the boss, the pay, each other. I open the door again and say, "It's been an hour."

"Dr. Miller is running behind."

"I understand that happens. Believe me, I understand, but someone needs to reassure the patients that they aren't being ignored."

Shortly my oncologist rushes into the room, apologizing for the delay.

"I really, really understand, Ben, that doctors get tied up; it's a regular occurrence in my clinic. But when that happens, the staff needs to communicate the situation to the patients."

He agrees and apparently feels the need to justify the delay, because he says, "One of my patients has a recurrence of her cancer and had many good questions that needed to be answered. She's an executive for DaimlerChrysler and. . . ." He pauses a moment and then continues, ". . . she's probably the smartest patient I've ever had."

My ego has been pierced, has instantly deflated. It lies on the floor in a little shriveled pile. To myself I say, "I thought *I* was your smartest patient."

He was speaking to the doctor me, sharing this vignette as a medical colleague. I heard it, however, as the patient me, the one who wants her physician's undivided attention, to be special in his eyes, to be the smartest. What he really meant was that his other patient is the most beautiful apple in the apple crate, which should have no relevance to me because I'm an orange.

In my journal, I write:

> *The mournful sound of a distant train breaks the quiet of the night. The railroad tracks pass through town about a mile from here, on the old rail bed that parallels the Huron River. The tracks ride the stone causeway over Fleming Creek and cross Dixboro Road at the automatic semaphore. As the train races through the dark, the*

*engineer sets off the warning signal. Its wail is comforting, familiar, full of soul.*

⚘

I'm standing in the hallway of the Cancer Center, waiting for the elevator. One of the pediatric doctors walks over to the wall and pushes the "up" button. With his arms folded across his chest, he stares at the numbers as they light up, one by one, above the elevator door: 6 . . . 5 . . . 4.

"Don . . . ," I say to him.

He turns, a question on his face.

"I'm Janet Gilsdorf." This man and I have worked in the children's hospital since I arrived in Ann Arbor eighteen years ago. Today I'm a stranger to him.

"Oh, yes . . . Janet." He smiles. "How're you doing?"

"I look different than I used to so I introduce myself to old friends."

"Oh, of course." He shakes his head. "I recognize you. I was just distracted." We both know that his comment was a little white lie, and it hangs in the silent air between us like a bad smell.

⚘

It's five days after Thanksgiving, and I have just climbed out of my "cradle" for the last time.

"Do you want to save it?" one of the technicians asks.

"No."

I say good-bye to the technicians, extending my best wishes to the one who is getting married soon and my encouragement to the one who is building a new house. I walk out the door. I don't *ever* have to sit in that waiting room again. After many long months, I'm done, *really finished*, with the entire cancer treatment.

It's an ending, the thing I don't do well. Rather than feeling jubilant, I'm weary, depleted, as empty as a cave. And it's a long way back to my real life.

I've been invited to give Pediatric Grand Rounds at the University of Minnesota next week; another airplane ride, another presentation in my wig. I need to finish making my slides.

As I round the corner to my office, I stop. A giant, crimson helium balloon floats in front of my door, tethered to the knob. Written in loopy script across the balloon are the words "You're awesome." As soon as she sees me, Renee, our secretary, gathers the staff, faculty, and fellows to celebrate the completion of my treatment. Renee serves homemade coffee cake and Amy, our administrator, presents me with a gift—Dr. Seuss's book *Oh, the Places You'll Go.*

Amy suggests I read it out loud. Standing in my doorway, I read this children's book to my infectious diseases colleagues who lean against the walls in the hall, balancing their paper plates loaded with cake and their Styrofoam cups full of coffee. As I recite the brilliant, zany, soaring rhymes of Dr. Seuss, I try to be animated, to express with my voice the vitality of the book. "Today is your day. You're off to great places! You're off and away!" As the words fly out of me, their layered meanings speak of new beginnings. I fear I might cry. I take a deep breath and continue reading.

This ending is the final chapter in the book of my cancer, or at least the treatment section of that book. The finality is dizzying. A part of me clings to the cancer; its ending, after all, is still a loss. This disease has been central to my being, has guided my every thought and action, for over nine months, ironically the gestational period of a new human life. And, after this ending, then what? Another beginning? Leading where?

THREE / Reentry and Beyond

# CHAPTER 17

Emerging

*My choices hang in the closet* before me: the old charcoal blazer plus the concrete-colored skirt that brushes my ankles *or* the new burgundy pantsuit. Which should I wear today? Tomorrow? Forever?

When I first ordered my cancer wardrobe my friend Emmy predicted it would become a living metaphor. She's a prophet, for my new clothes mirror what I expect of my life since cancer: comfort, color, tuned in, open to unexpected adventures.

Now that I'm free from the prison of cancer treatment, I'm eager to move on. I want to jettison the old in favor of the new. In this fresh, free world, I'll throw open the doors that have no locks and gaze out at meadows that have no fences. I'll walk tall in the sunshine.

I choose the burgundy pantsuit. The gray gabardine skirt and charcoal flannel blazer go into the box for the Purple Heart Charities.

"We have two new consults," the pediatric infectious diseases fellow says, "one on 7 West—a thirteen-year-old, three months post–stem cell transplant, with fever and a new pulmonary infiltrate—and the other on 5W—a six-year-old with fever and limp, probably osteomyelitis. Should we see the new ones first or the old ones?"

It's my third week of attending on the Pediatric Infectious Diseases consult service. On January 1 I returned to full-time clinical work, and I'm exhausted. Every evening I drag myself home, eat dinner with Jim, and vegetate in my chair until I can stay awake no longer. My brain doesn't work right yet; its gears are sluggish and off-center.

*MSSA, MRSA, MRSE, beta-lactamase positive, mecA negative.* When these words roll past me I have to stop a moment to grab the concepts they convey.

But, being back is good, returns me to where I belong. As I walk the halls of the children's hospital, I feel the history of the place: the infectious diseases ward that used to be on 7 West and our offices at the end of the corridor; nurses who have moved on; students and residents, graduated long ago, who are now successful doctors; the patient with cutaneous coccidiomycosis whom a resident described in the *Journal of Pediatric Infectious Diseases;* the patient with cefotaxime-resistant *Streptococcus pneumoniae* meningitis, one of the first reported in the United States, also written up by a resident. So many, many patients. So many, many trainees. These memories are like silver polish as they rub away the tarnish of my yearlong absence and restore the shine of being a pediatrician and educator.

"Dr. Gilsdorf." One of the residents stops me in the hall. "Remember that patient with septic arthritis last week?"

"Yes."

"Well, his father said the cutest thing. He said, 'You know that lady doctor with the hat?'"

He was talking about one of my winter hats, the brown felt cloche with Hoffman Hackles from Cabela's sporting goods store pinned to the side. I have thought the feathers elegant in the way they sway and bounce when I walk.

"He said, 'That hat . . . it's sooooo Ann Arbor.'"

I'm horrified. Somehow I expected that patients and their families wouldn't notice the hat. What did he mean? Did he see its elegance? Maybe not. Maybe he equated it with Ann Arbor's reputation as a haughty, disgustingly arrogant place. I don't want to stand out as odd. I want to fit in to the background, to be another of the normal doctors here.

At my next oncology clinic appointment, I explain my fatigue to Ben.

"You're doing a whole month of service?" he asks.

"Yes, and it's killing me."

"Well, that's too much. In adult oncology we used to do a month at a time, but several years ago we changed to two-week stints. By the third week we were worn out and crabby and less attentive."

That's a great idea. This spring when I make up the schedule for the Pediatrics Infectious Diseases service, I'll offer the faculty two- or four-week shifts. I'll definitely choose the two-week option for myself.

Carl left our regular lab meeting early to attend a seminar in another department, so I'm on my own reviewing the week's experiments with the lab gang. Even though I attended the lab meetings whenever I could during my treatment, it feels as if I've been far away on a long, long trip. I need to catch up with what they're doing, need to focus harder on their experimental results and what they tell us.

Standing, I bend across the conference room table, my belly rubbing against its wooden surface, and examine Melinda's dot blots. We discuss the "edge effects" and how they may alter a positive signal. Graham suggests a change in the hybridization conditions. The results suggest that the membranes stuck together during the incubation so the enzyme didn't optimally reach the spots on the bottom sheet. I suggest additional control bacteria to include in the next assay. The spots on the membrane are lined up like rosy-gray checkers in eight rows and twelve columns. Once again I'm in charge of my research lab, capable of interpreting the data the technologists and students generate, able to guide them in designing the experiments. It's a slow start, but I'm on my way to becoming a fully functioning scientist again.

"What are we doing today?" Jane asks. This is my first visit to my hairdresser since she gave me the pixie cut when my hair was falling out. Her fingers comb the chalky kinks that grow on my head. Jim says it looks like someone glued dust bunnies all over my scalp.

"Oh, I don't know. What are the possibilities?" The kinks are too tight, but I'm very glad to have hair and very sick of being the oddball in the hats. I'm ready to go "bare" now.

"Well, we could shape it a little today, and as it grows out further, we can decide if you want to return to longer or keep it shorter. I suspect it will straighten out as it grows."

"Good, because I don't like the tight kinks. They remind me of my Grandma Nelson's bad home permanents."

Jane chuckles and begins to snip.

I'm in room 16 in our pediatric clinic, my stethoscope dangling from my neck. One of my patients, a ten-year-old boy with a chronic infection, is seated on the examining table. I've taken care of him for about five years, since a week after he arrived in America, sick. With my hand on the boy's shoulder, I explain the situation to his father, what might happen in the short run, what is inevitable in the long run.

Suddenly an epiphany—an awareness, a force, an energy—sweeps over me with laserlike intensity and clarity. At that moment, I'm more mindful of being a physician than I have ever been.

I stop talking and pat Brandon's shoulder. To myself I silently say, I'm *so* glad to be here. *So* glad to be your doctor. *So* glad to have the privilege to know you, to watch you grow up, to be a part of your life. I'm elated to be standing beside this examining table rather than sitting on the stiff paper in a hospital gown.

For a piece I'm writing, I need to know the name of the University of Connecticut's hometown. I know it starts with an *S* and think it ends with an *s*. What's in between? The chemo has knotted the mental connections I need to recall this fact. On the blackboard of my mind, I search for the word, placing a capital *S* at the left and a lowercase *s* at the right. Suddenly the middle letters fly into place, *t . . . o . . . r . . . r*, and I read the word. Storrs. That's it.

The study coordinator from the School of Nursing, the lady who administered the tests to document my level of goofiness while receiving chemotherapy, pokes her head into the doorway of my office.

"Good. You're here," she says. I offer her a seat. "I have the final report of your testing." My scores didn't change much over the course of the treatment, except that both my arm and leg muscle strength steadily decreased.

"That's probably because I'm in horrible shape. My muscles turned to mush."

"Well, you have been pretty inactive . . ."

"I still think the tests weren't sensitive enough to capture my brain dysfunction," I say, interrupting her. "It might have been subtle, but it was very, very real."

She turns toward my miniature chair collection on the file cabinet. She seems to be changing the subject.

"Nice office," she says. Her eyes stop on the Red Rose tea figurines, then on the antique wood and glass encased balance I rescued from the microbiology laboratory trash bin. "But you need something living in here. Maybe a plant."

On the way home I stop at Busch's grocery store and buy a philodendron.

This morning I arrange the plant beside my desk, setting it on an old wooden stand from our basement. It's lovely. The nurse was right. My office needed vitality, something growing, something green, something to enliven the space around me.

⚛

As Esther approaches, her body is outlined by daylight that streams through the glass doors of the hospital's entryway. I haven't seen her for a long time, not since before my cancer. A senior physician and well beyond age seventy, she doesn't look a day older now than she did eighteen years ago when I first met her.

She stops to chat, to catch up. I explain that I've been lying low because of breast cancer. She nods. Then she lists her acquaintances who recently have had cancer: Clarise with colon cancer, Diana with lung cancer, Maureen with a lymphoma. She speaks in the same matter-of-fact manner she would use to recite her most recent travels.

What does the world look like to someone who is approaching eighty years old? She's watched poor health engulf her friends, one after the other. I suppose she's resigned to the fact that she may be the next to fall, that illness and death come to everyone in good time, and that the older you are, the closer the axe blade.

Esther's easy acceptance of cancer among her friends depresses me. I want her to rail against it, to yell and scream at the unfairness of it all, to loudly proclaim that I'm too young for this terrible disease.

I don't want Esther to regard my cancer as the obvious first stop on my road to the end. My expectation, after all, is that, since I have completed the year of therapy, I will soon be back to my old self, and by that I mean my twenty-five-year-old self. I won't be satisfied to go back to my fifty-five-year-old self with its stiff joints, limited endurance, dampened passion, raging cynicism; to its diminished enthusiasm for a big, totally new endeavor such as building a mission hospital in the Congo or orbiting Mars with a NASA crew. I want to return to the ambitions and lofty goals of my twenty-five-year-old self, and since I've passed through cancer, I believe I've earned that privilege, even if it defies all laws of thermo-, hydro-, electro-, and psychodynamics.

Esther continues down the hall, her back straight as a yardstick, a bounce in her gait, only a few gray hairs on her head.

Our clinic coordinator, two medical students, a resident, four infectious diseases fellows, and four faculty crowd into the staff room. Some discuss a patient's diagnostic workup or response to treatment; others scroll through a patient's electronic chart or read medical information on the computerized library. John gazes at the view box as Jason points the tip of his pen to a white patch on all four x-ray films, two postero-anterior views, two lateral. The patches on the most recent films are smaller than those on the earlier ones. That's good.

Alex quizzes the students with infectious diseases questions. It's noisy. I glance at the marker board beneath the clock; four patients have been put in examining rooms, and three more wait in the reception area.

"OK, guys." My voice cuts through the din. All eyes turn toward me. "We have to speed up. We can't keep the patients waiting this long." Recollections of the Cancer Center swirl through my head: the registration desk, the reception area, the vital signs station, the examining room. The waiting. The waiting.

"Chris," I say to the clinic coordinator, "any possibility of additional rooms?"

"I'll check."

"I'll see the Edmund child now," I tell her. Two other patients on the board are mine. "While you're scouting up more rooms, please poke your head into rooms 14 and 17 and tell the Andersons and the Danforths we'll be in as soon as we can."

I turn to the resident beside me. "We don't want those poor folks to worry that they'll still be cooped up in that room—waiting—into next week."

George, our first-year fellow, is ready to tell me about DeShawna Edmund, a two-year-old who was sent to see us by her doctor because of a possible immune disorder. In the staff room, against the background racket, he describes the child's two episodes of pneumonia, her many ear infections. He details the family history, the review of systems, the laboratory tests the family doctor has already done. He shows me DeShawna's growth chart and describes the physical examination. We agree on a diagnostic workup, assuming my discussion with her parents and examination of their daughter don't point us in a different direction.

I knock on the door to the examining room and open it carefully to avoid striking DeShawna, in case she is near. Peering around the door's edge I locate the little girl, seated safely on her mother's lap. I haven't met the Edmunds yet, as their daughter is a new patient to our clinic.

"I'm Doctor Gilsdorf," I tell DeShawna's parents as I extend my hand to them. My encounter with the rude pathologist who biopsied my breast a year ago hovers in this room like a phantom.

Mr. and Mrs. Edmund introduce themselves and shake my hand.

Staring into their faces, first one, then the other, I add, "Sorry to keep you waiting."

They smile and answer in unison, "Oh, that's all right."

Months ago, while under the grip of Adriamycin and Cytoxan, I often thought about my medical colleagues and wrote those reflections, disjointed as they were, in my journal. I jotted down remembrances of us as scared, fumbling freshmen in the gross anatomy dissection laboratory, together memorizing every nerve, muscle, blood vessel, bone, ligament, and tendon in the human body. I recalled the camaraderie with which we faced heart-wrenching human tragedies that we'd never imagined possible. I remembered the crushing burden of responsibilities we weren't prepared for. Together we learned the reverence of a life ending, the awe of a life beginning.

While lying in my bed and nauseous from chemo, I recorded the quiet knowing with which my colleagues reacted to my cancer. I wrote of the beauty of our medical language—the timeless Latin words that rumble like wooden carts through the ages; the respectful eponyms that pay homage to the scientists of yore who first recognized the diseases; the modern, high-tech lingo that vibrates like the molecules it describes; rhythmic, tongue-twisting syllables such as *Zollinger-Ellison* and *cor pulmonale, Burkholderia cepacia* and *situs inversus, Fontan procedure* and *nuclear magnetic resonance.* I wrote of the efficiency with which these lovely utterances convey complicated meaning, of the ease with which their familiar phrases permit me to share the details of my illness with my colleagues.

Now I return to those journal entries to craft an anthem to my fellow physicians in honor of their kindness and understanding. I try to write the essay in first person, but it reads like a sappy, self-serving manifesto. I delete that version and rewrite it in the third person, past tense, hoping to distance myself from the woman with cancer, a woman known only as "she" in the essay. This is better. Maybe my cancer is still too recent, too raw, for me to embrace the woman as me. I need it to be "her" story, not mine.

After many edits, after input from my writers' group, after valuable suggestions from Jim, and following a fight with a computer virus, my essay is finally done. I send it to the *Journal of the American Medical Association*, for the "Piece of My Mind" section.

Several weeks later an envelope bearing the *JAMA* logo arrives in my mailbox. I'm afraid to read the message inside, can't bear for my essay to be rejected. I carry the envelope around the house for several hours and finally, in a fit of resignation, rip it open. The journal has accepted my essay.

On the day of publication, an e-mail arrives from the National Institutes of Health, from a woman who used to be on the university faculty. Her message tells of the ways my words moved her.

The e-mails and letters and phone calls keep coming and coming—from a high school classmate who is now a pediatrician, from an infectious diseases colleague who herself has just been diagnosed with breast cancer, from university faculty and staff, from medical school and high school classmates, from many strangers. It's overwhelming.

I learn about fifty-five-word stories from a writing magazine. They intrigue me. While crisp and instantly to the point, they possess all the elements of a short story: character, place, time, movement. I give it a try.

AT THE DELI
by Janet R. Gilsdorf

*A year ago in this store, the red-headed deli clerk looked into my pale face framed by a green silk scarf and said, "Oh . . . I had cancer, too."*

*Today, as I scoop Spanish olives into a plastic container, Johnny Mathis begins to sing from far, far away: "And I say to myself, 'It's wonderful, wonderful . . .'"*

# Chapter 18

It Never Goes Away

*A lump appears in my right breast,* the good one. To me it feels exactly like the left-sided almond that was my first cancer.

Jim feels it, thinks it needs to be investigated.

My radiation oncologist feels it. She isn't worried but orders an ultrasound anyway. It's normal.

Jim isn't convinced. "I'd be more comfortable if a surgeon felt that."

"Jim, I'm satisfied with the evaluation I've had." My voice is edgy with frustration.

"Well, I'm not." He calls my surgeon and sets up an appointment for me.

I'm furious with Jim. He's treating me like a child.

Although I feel like a hypochondriac, I keep the appointment with my surgeon. Myron reviews the ultrasound, examines my breast, and says, "It's soft, feels like a cystic duct. I don't think we need to do anything."

Jim settles down.

It's three o'clock in the morning, and I can't sleep. For the past two weeks my left wrist has hurt. At first I disregarded the pain, calling it arthritis. I've had arthritis in my hips and toes for years but never in my arms or hands. I turn on the light, read the short story in the latest *New Yorker,* turn off the light, and toss and turn. Jim sleeps beside me, oblivious to my worries. Then, on the view box inside my closed eyelids, I see, for the eighth night running, an x-ray of my left hand. The metacarpals splay like a bony fan. The carpals are stacked, three deep, in each finger. Something is wrong. The navicular bone isn't normal. Smack in its center is a lytic lesion, a hole the size of a pea where cells from metastatic breast cancer are chewing away the bone.

A week later, at my clinic appointment, I describe the pain to my oncologist.

"You're worried about a recurrence. I can tell." He bends and twists my wrist, palpates my joint.

"Uh-huh."

He reassures me that metastases from the breast never, or almost never, appear below the knee or beyond the elbow. "It's probably your arthritis."

The imaginary x-ray of a metastatic wrist lesion goes away. Eventually the pain goes away too.

Will it ever end? My treatment is over, but will I ever be confident that the cancer won't come back? Breast cancer isn't like lymphoma, where five years' survival pretty much means long-term cure. Breast cancer can reappear, in a bone, the brain, the lung, or the liver, ten . . . twenty years later.

"When do you suppose I'll get the brain scan, chest x-ray, bone scan, and abdominal CT?" I ask Jim.

"What for?"

"To detect metastases."

"The answer is 'never.'"

"Never? Why not?" I'm dumbfounded. "Don't we want to find them early?"

"Doesn't matter," Jim says. "The mortality rate for metastatic breast cancer is the same whether it's detected early or late."

I nod. At least now I know.

"What's wrong with your hand?" Amanda, one of my patients, asks as I approach her with my stethoscope. Like many other five year olds she zooms immediately to the core of a matter. She has spotted the compression garment on my left wrist and palm, the fingerless elastic mitten that hopefully controls my lymphedema.

"Hush," her mother whispers, slipping her fingers over her daughter's mouth.

"Oh, it's a little sore." I massage the pressure glove that encircles my puffy hand. "It'll be better real soon."

Amanda shrugs and pulls up her shirt so I can examine her chest.

It's right on schedule. Four o'clock in the afternoon and my cheeks flush. A river of sweat trickles down my breastbone. A wave of heat sears my skin as if I'm standing downwind from a prairie fire. It always comes in the late afternoon, but it also comes during the night, in the morning, in the evening, pretty much anytime. It's a tamoxiphen rush, a feverish surge similar to a perimenopausal hot flash. I tolerate this better than I did the hot flashes. These rushes may be every bit as disruptive, but they have a higher calling, for they are a side effect of tamoxiphen. This drug contains a hormonelike molecule that will block my natural estrogens from docking to the estrogen receptors on my cancer cells. If I take it for five years, the probability of my developing recurrent breast cancer may be reduced by 25 percent. By my calculations, the benefit is large enough to put up with the rushes, no matter how frequent.

The pain in my right hip, the sensation of bugs crawling over my left shoulder, the momentary out-of-body lapses that fold over me from time to time, the cough that lasts for weeks, the muscle spasm in my left neck. Are they metastases? I try to ignore them. But, it isn't wise to ignore them completely. I need to pay attention to my body, to notice signals that something might be wrong.

So, is it smart to ignore the drenching sweats after a long walk? What about my fatigue when climbing steps? Are these the signs of heart failure, the end result of Adriamycin cardiac toxicity further aggravated by radiation over the left side of my chest?

I dump all these symptoms, like a bushel of bananas, in my oncologist's lap, as if to say, "Here. Sort through these. Find the rotten ones."

❧

We're at thirty-seven thousand feet, somewhere over South Dakota on our way to Portland, Oregon, to visit Dan and Bean. I'm cold. It's October, and I'm dressed in head-to-toe wool, so this chill makes no sense. As I turn my attention from the novel in my lap to my body's thermal state, I realize I'm not freezing all over. Rather, only my left arm is cold; it feels as if it's submerged in a bucket of ice water, achingly cold and wet. I run my right hand under the sleeve of my sweater, under my compression garment, and up and down my left arm. The skin feels warm and dry from the outside. From the inside, it's still frigid and damp.

What's going on now? It's been a year and a half since my surgery. The fingers of my left hand aren't blue, aren't cold. I feel my left radial pulse. It's normal, so my brachial artery must still be feeding blood to that arm. Maybe, when the cabin pressure is lower than the atmospheric pressure in Ann Arbor, the compression sleeve is too tight. I've been warned that air travel makes lymphedemic arms swell. I guess it's possible the lymphedema is worsening now, since the lymphatic drainage system through my chest has been further damaged by fibrosis—scars—after radiation.

I pull off the elastic compression sleeve. Doesn't help at all. I consult Jim. He feels my fingers, my pulse, the skin of my left arm. He also has no idea what's going on. I pull my left arm out of the sleeve of my sweater and cradle it against my warm tummy. Doesn't help. Jim wraps my chest and left arm in a Northwest Airlines blanket. Doesn't help. I return to my novel but can't concentrate from the bone-chilling cold.

Somewhere over western Oregon, the cold disappears.

A month later the cold returns when I clasp my watch around my left wrist. I blame the cool metal of the watchband.

A month after that, I'm curled in my easy chair, reading, when the cold returns—same sensation of my left arm dangling in a bucket of ice water. Same warm fingers, normal pulse, warm skin from the outside.

Soon it happens at least once a week.

Now it happens several times a day and lasts from ten minutes to several hours. I suspect it's set off by air blowing on me. Also seems worse in damp weather. My compression sleeve appears to have nothing to do with the cold; leaving it on or taking it off makes no difference. Around the house I wear half a sweater, my left arm swaddled in both sleeves, one inside the other.

The cold disturbs me while reading or writing and is less noticeable when I'm distracted by conversation. Sometimes I find myself in a thermal muddle; my body is overheated from the tamoxiphen rushes, and my left arm is freezing. Finally I tell my oncologist.

He feels my fingers, my pulse, the skin of my left arm.

"It doesn't feel cold now," I say, "but even when it does, the skin is warm."

He pounds up and down my backbone and watches for my reaction. "Does that hurt?"

"No."

He's testing for a metastasis in my spine.

"I think it's a paresthesia left over from my axillary dissection," I say, giving him my explanation for the cold. "Probably, the severed nerve ends in my brachial plexus are trying to reconnect." I wiggle my fingers against each other to illustrate my theory. "And they are all tangled up. The timing after my operation seems about right for that."

He nods and scratches his head. "Could be. I want to make sure it's not vascular. We'll get a Doppler of your brachial artery to be sure it's not compromised."

"Not compromised" is what he said. He's still searching for a metastasis, one that might be pinching off part of the blood supply to that arm.

So I have the Doppler study first and then visit the vascular surgeon.

"Normal," the surgeon says. "I think your paresthesia idea is probably right."

My left breast, the one that had the cancer, starts to ache. I figure the irradiated tissues are still healing and rearranging themselves through scarring, even though it's been nearly two years since I finished radiation. But today I examine that breast, something I've not done regularly because the anatomy is so distorted that all I feel is shelves of scar tissue.

This time there's a lump, the size of a marble, below the nipple. It's discrete and firm, standing out like a boulder from the surrounding soft breast tissue and the scar tissue above.

Jim examines my breast. He throws his arms about my shoulders and chokes into my neck, "That is very worrisome." When he composes himself, he adds, "More so, even, than your first lump. It should be needled."

His reaction scares me. He's supposed to be the reassuring one, the voice of reason that dampens my fears, the purveyor of common sense to balance my overinterpretation of what's happening in my body.

The next morning I phone my radiation oncologist and explain the new lump. She tells me she'll get right back to me. A half hour later, she calls again to say she has spoken with Art Young; Myron, my old oncologic surgeon, has moved to Texas so he can't deal with this. She has set up an appointment for the new surgeon to see me the next day.

Art examines my breast. "Pretty soft," he says of the mass. "We won't go sticking needles in you without imaging studies." He hands me an x-ray requisition. "So, go to radiology and get a mammogram and ultrasound. I'll see you back in the clinic afterwards."

The mammogram, with extra films using a smaller paddle that grinds like an alligator wrench on my already painful, irradiated breast, is normal. During the ultrasound I watch the shadows on the monitor, not knowing what I'm looking at. The radiologist drives the gelled probe up and down and around my breast. "There's a spot here, where that lump is." She sets her finger on a small gray blur on the monitor. "It might be scar tissue. I can't tell for sure. I'll call Art and discuss this with him."

My heart races, and I feel faint. The scar from my old lumpectomy is nowhere near this new mass. What's she talking about? Radiation scarring?

The next year of my life marches through my mind. Mastectomy. Chemo again? What kind? Any residual tumor would, most likely, be resistant to the Adriamycin and Cytoxan and Taxol I had before. Will I lose my hair again? I know I gave my wig to the Purple Heart Charities, but I think I still have some of my straw hats and many of the flowers Barb made for them.

I don't want to go through all that again. I'll quit work. I'll just give up. I'll go to bed and cuddle under my blankets forever.

Art walks into the examining room with a tray of supplies. "I doubt this is anything to worry about, but because of the ultrasound abnormality, we'll do an aspirate."

He injects a dot of Lidocaine into my skin over the lump. The local anesthetic stings, but I don't feel the aspiration needle at all. It's over so fast that I assume he made only one pass, unlike the four passes into my unanesthetized breast the last time. Every doctor does the procedure differently, but this time it's more comfortable. I hope he obtained enough tissue for a valid sample during that one pass of the needle.

Two days later he sends me an e-mail.

```
From: Arthur Young
To: janetgils@umich.edu
Date: July 20, 2002 4:34:23 PM
Subject: Tried to reach you by phone but got no
answer. The aspirate shows a few glandular cells
and no malignancy. I wouldn't pursue this any fur-
ther.
```

I'm relieved. So is Jim. I don't know if I should stop examining my breasts or not; I can't seem to tell what's important.

My nephew in Texas is getting married, and I need a new outfit for the wedding. Rows of garments hang before me on the display racks in Letty's dress shop.

I pull out the pretty blue one, hold it against my body, and step to the mirror. The azure color makes my eyes come alive. The crepe fabric is soft and drapey. This dress, however, won't work. It has short sleeves. The compression garment on my left arm will show, and I'll look bionic. Maybe I could leave the compression sleeve off during the wedding and the reception.

No, I have to wear the sleeve. My arm feels funny—heavy, achy, numb—without it. The elastic sleeve seems to dissipate the weirdness that I feel; it's the same counterirritant principle as white noise. In addition, the skin of that arm is ghostly pale while the hand is nicely sun-kissed. A tan line wraps around my left wrist.

I reach for a satin dress, the one the color of the lilacs in our front yard. It has long sleeves. In the dressing room, I slip it over my head and confront the mirror. My gaze moves immediately to my chest. The off-kilter nipples—one higher, one lower—lift the smooth, mauve fabric awkwardly. As far as breasts are concerned, symmetry is normal, is expected, is beautiful. If I get this dress I'll have to cover the top with a jacket.

I wish I could see my body as others might—as a memorial to the wonders of the medical treatments that rid me of my cancer; as yet another imperfect entity in this imperfect but good enough world; as a biologic variant, surgically crafted. Instead I see it as mutilated. Disfigured. Ugly. And it's mine for the rest of my life.

A dream: I'm a student taking a final exam. There's only one question—compose a paragraph.

I can't do it. On my legal pad I write a couple sentences and then scratch them out. I write another few sentences and then scratch them out, too. Over and over, write and scratch it out. Write and scratch it out.

My instructor sees that I'm having trouble and brings me a computer. Still I can't write anything that's satisfactory. I type a couple sentences and then delete. Over and over, type and delete. Type and delete. The rest of the students have completed their exam paragraph, and I'm still struggling. I fret. I worry. I panic. Nothing of value gets written.

Then I wake up. The irony of the dream keeps me up the rest of the night—I couldn't complete my exam question; I can't forget the cancer.

# CHAPTER 19

*The Road to Wellness Goes through*
*Monterey, California*
*and Almaty, Kazakhstan*

*Now that I've finished my cancer therapy,* Michigan seems like a box around me. Its walls crush my sides; its top hangs low over my head. The air inside, still and stale, smells of lingering illness.

I'm furious at the current mess in the medical system; upset that, for lack of money, patients can't get the basic care they need; angry that physicians have been herded with economic whips into systems that seem to serve administrators and third-party payers rather than ill people; frustrated with the layers of bureaucracy that separate doctors from their patients. .

I need a break from this sea of sickness, from the vise of health-care administration; I need to think creative thoughts and take on something new. I fidget. I squirm. I seethe. When I look at my wish list I see simplicity, beauty, wellness. I reach out to seize these wishes, but they slip like oil through my fingers. Maybe if I move a little, if I change my position on the planet, I can connect with them. But how?

In the past, working with profoundly sick children didn't bother me. But, the added weight of my own illness, whose specter still loiters in the corners of every room and still casts long shadows over my future, saps me. I'm completely uninsulated against my patients' discomforts; I want to yank out the nasogastric tubes that irritate their noses, want to quit drawing blood, stop starting IVs. I look into their blank, hopeless faces and ask myself, "What are we doing here? Are we giving them precious life or delaying a merciful death?" Being a patient and physician in the same place at the same time—dishing it out and getting it simultaneously, riding the thick wall that separates medical caregivers from those they serve—is too much.

An op-ed piece in the *New York Times* supports a policy to give every American the smallpox vaccine as protection against a possible bioterrorism attack. I'm appalled that this nonsense appears in a reputable newspaper. The author is a biologist, an educator, a scientific gadfly. He is neither a physician nor a public health professional. He has never injected biologic material into a child's buttock, has no notion of the risk-benefit calculations that every physician runs before subjecting a patient to a medical treatment or diagnostic test or immunization. He has never seen vaccinia, a sometimes fatal consequence of the smallpox vaccine, has never stared in disbelief at its oozing ulcers that dissolve a person's skin, all the while knowing he caused it to happen. He has never looked into the questioning, imploring, desperate-to-trust eyes of a mother and assured her that what he is about to do to her most precious treasure, her child, is absolutely right. This guy doesn't know what he's talking about.

At the same time, a new interest has found me. I'm fascinated with the ease by which scientific methods can be used to engineer bacteria and viruses into anything a microbiologist may design. The tools to transform microbes are taught to biology students around the world; every liberal arts college in America and research university across the globe has laboratories in which these experiments can be done. Moving genes in and out of bacteria and viruses is the lifeblood of biomedical research. It's the way new treatments are constructed, new diagnostic tests are developed, new knowledge about all things biologic is generated. Yet, these powerful scientific tools could be misused by unscrupulous individuals to construct microbial weapons.

In the car on the way to work, I hear an interview with Jonathan Tucker from the Center for Nonproliferation Studies at the Monterey Institute of International Studies (MIIS). Jonathan has written several books on bioterrorism. The next day I hear an interview with Raymond Zilinskas, a microbiologist and former weapons inspector in Iraq, also at MIIS.

As they speak, I remember the MIIS signs during our visits with Joe in Monterey. When we drove past its low-slung, California-style buildings—flags of the world flapping from the roof, lush coastal blooms concealing the foundation—I asked Joe, "What's that?"

"The Monterey Institute."

"Right. What do they do there?"

"It's a language school."

From the Internet I discover it's also a foreign affairs graduate school that houses the Center for Nonproliferation Studies.

These seemingly unrelated thoughts—the medical mess, the threat of microbial weapons, the MIIS, the outrageous op-ed by an uninformed person—shuffle together in my mind like a deck of cards during my Grandpa Nelson's cribbage games. One slaps against another. They divide, half into the right side, half into the left. They fold together again into a single pile but in a newfound order this time. Different ideas, like the cards, touch each other now; yet different ones touch after the next shuffle. The cards are dealt, and when they are picked up and spread into a fan, one word emerges—*sabbatical.*

I've never taken a sabbatical leave, though as a tenured professor at the university, I've been eligible for one for about fifteen years. My lab, my patients, my administrative and teaching responsibilities, and my family—especially when the kids were younger—have kept me riveted to Ann Arbor. Taking a sabbatical at my university, an alternative to going away, would be an exercise in frustration of enormous proportions. I would be away but not away. The phone would still ring, e-mails would clog my computer, my pager would still beep. The old commitments would tug at me, my hyper-responsible self would cave in to the demands.

But, something is different now. The breath of mortality blew on my face and nothing bad happened. The chain that ties me to my work has become elastic, its links are less rigid as they spin on a newfound swivel.

The notion of a sabbatical won't go away. It becomes the solution to my every irritation. I'm cranky about the operation of the clinic and think "sabbatical." I'm frustrated with the difficulty in getting an MRI for a patient and think "sabbatical." I'm offended at having to justify to an insurance bureaucrat the use of an expensive antibiotic to treat a resistant germ and think "sabbatical."

In a spurt of mischief that, in my view, borders on recklessness, I send off an e-mail to Jonathan Tucker inquiring about opportunities for visiting scientists at the institute. By return e-mail, he reminds me that he is in the Washington office and refers me to Ray in the California office. For a moment I consider a sabbatical in Washington, D.C., but in the next click of my office clock's second hand, I send off an e-mail to Ray. I want to go to Monterey, want to escape the never-ending sickness that smothers me in Michigan, want to be surrounded by wellness and warmth and endless beauty—in California.

A week later, Claire and I walk to lunch at the Borders bookstore in downtown Ann Arbor. After we settle beside our shared sandwich and wedge of blueberry pie, I pull a sheet of paper, fresh off my office printer, from my purse.

"Listen to this and tell me what you think." I read out loud. "The Center for Nonproliferation Studies at the Monterey Institute of International Studies announces the availability of fellowship positions. Those interested in the Chemical and Biologic Weapons Program are especially encouraged to apply."

"Do it," Claire says.

"Really?"

"Apply today."

"What about my lab, my patients, my students, my division . . ." The old responsibility noose slinks back into my reasoning, the whiney refrain of martyrdom into my voice.

"They'll get over it," she says. "You need to go."

Before leaving work for the day, I apply. Several weeks later MIIS accepts me as a senior visiting scientist. I apply for a fellowship award from the National Institutes of Health to support my sabbatical (even though the university will pay my full salary for six months or half salary for twelve months). The NIH money will help defray my travel and living expenses. The grant application, entitled "The Two-Edged Sword: Vaccine Technology and Biological Weapons," receives the lowest (which, as in golf, is best) score I have ever received from the NIH. Obviously the topic scared the bejesus out of the reviewers.

After weighing the options, a six-month sabbatical seems best. My husband can't abandon his one-doctor surgical practice to go with me. I design the Pediatric Infectious Diseases schedule so that my clinical obligations for the entire year will be fulfilled within the six months before I leave.

Everything is set. MIIS will clear out an office for me, and they have given me passwords to their computer system. Through the Internet I have rented a furnished apartment a half block from the bay. Jim will drive with me to Monterey (so I can have my car there) and fly back to Ann Arbor; six months later he will do the trip in reverse. The plane tickets are purchased.

Three weeks before our planned departure, I walk into our bedroom as my husband undresses for bed.

"What is that?" I point to the wires taped to his bare chest.

"A Holter monitor."

"What on earth for?"

"Well, my heart's been doing flip-flops, so Marek"—the cardiologist who shares office space with Jim—"wants to see a twenty-four-hour tracing."

"In the future, Jim, tell me these things." Maybe he's trying to shield me from more medical worry. Nice thought, but I'd rather have the facts.

After reading the tracing, which shows Jim's heartbeat to be wildly irregular, Marek orders an ECHO cardiogram, a stress test, and, finally, a coronary artery angiogram.

In the darkened cardiac catherization suite Marek and I hover over the computerized x-ray images of my husband's heart while, down the hall, Jim sleeps off his sedation.

"See the obstruction here?" Marek stabs the point of a pen at one of the white branching squiggles on the computer screen. "And here. And here."

He calls the cardiovascular surgeon, and they discuss the possibilities. In the end, the only real option is a CABG—coronary artery bypass graft, or *cabbage* in medical lingo.

"We'll do it on Monday," Marek tells me. Today is Friday. As we speak, my sabbatical disintegrates and disappears into the realm of improbability.

"No, don't," Jim says when I suggest canceling my sabbatical. "It's a great opportunity for you. I'll be fine."

Jim's heart surgery goes well. To see him through the early postoperative recovery period, I delay my start time at MIIS by a couple weeks.

"You know, Jim," I say, desperately trying to keep my sabbatical alive and starting to plan for it again, "you can recover from the surgery while riding in the front seat of my car just as easily as sitting in your La-Z-Boy. After that, you'll be up to the airplane ride home from California."

He agrees.

Shortly before our next date to leave Michigan, Jim has another bout of irregular heartbeat and drives himself to the emergency room in the middle of the night because I'm at a bioterrorism conference in Washington, D.C. By the time I learn of it, he's been admitted to the hospital and has been cardioverted, his heartbeat is regular again, and he's ready to drive himself back home.

A week later, the irregular heartbeat returns. It goes away with the help of expensive, new wonder drugs, which Jim calls his "preservatives." Finally Marek sets us straight.

"Jim," he says, "I think a cross-country road trip, especially through the relatively uninhabited western states, isn't wise at this time."

"Honey," I say, my heart broken at the possible loss of my sabbatical, "Marek's right. Your going with me to California would be stupid."

"Maybe you could drive yourself or fly and rent a car out there. Don't cancel your sabbatical because of me."

When my sister Nancy learns of my plight, she offers to drive with me. "Give me a week to rearrange my life here in Portland."

I'm still reluctant to leave. Jim's health is somewhat tenuous, although his heart is now beating in a regular rhythm. What kind of wife leaves her husband in such a state? Jim insists he'll be fine and that I should go. Turns out Joe is coming home on leave from the navy for three weeks and can be Jim's companion and errand boy. Nancy and I arrange to depart the day before Joe is to arrive—the fourth in a series of ever-later departure dates.

We're driving across the salt flats of Utah; I'm at the wheel. Nothing grows here. Absolutely nothing. Grit the color of coconut meat covers the ground to the horizon, broken only by railroad tracks that parallel the highway. Occasional messages, such as "Ed loves Ellen," are spelled out in black stones on the chalky earth. For three days, Nancy and I have sat eighteen inches apart in the front seat of my new PT Cruiser.

I glance at my sister, at her face in profile against the desolate Utah terrain that flies past the car window, at the threads of silver in her dark coffee-colored hair, at the way a curl twists with abandon along her neck, at the wrinkles beside her eyes that deepen with her smile. Her right foot, wrapped in a red and yellow argyle sock, rests on the dashboard, and she studies the information she ordered from AAA. She's trying to locate a motel in Elko, Nevada, so we can have dinner at the Star, a Basque inn that caters to the local Spanish sheepherders. In her lap rests the travel log she's keeping, a detailed account of where we spend the nights and where we refuel, of gas mileage and restaurant expenses. My log of this trip, tucked in my overnight case, is my journal, in which I record my impressions of the scenery and the people, my imaginings, my perceptions.

Since leaving Ann Arbor (in a snowstorm) we have reminisced about our early lives together, and I'm more appreciative of her than ever before. We haven't always been good friends, but during this trip we have had no disagreements—no squabbles over when to stop, which way to turn, where to spend the night, whether to pull into the next Kentucky Fried Chicken joint (to satisfy a sudden craving of mine) or the next Taco Bell (to satisfy hers). Both my big-sister tendency to boss my little sister and her lifelong agitation at being bossed seem to have vanished. She herself had a coronary artery bypass operation at age fifty-five; I had cancer at age fifty-five. Our many differences seem inconsequential now.

I look at the set of her jaw, the same jaw as our Grandma Nelson. I look at her nose, our father's nose. She's a mother, a wife, a good friend to many people, an artist who focuses her creative energy on pottery. She's funny, imaginative, sharp tongued, determined. Right now the most endearing thing about my sister is her willingness to accompany me on this crazy adventure. I am escaping my work, my home, my friends, and my husband (who is still recovering from major heart surgery) for six months, and she is helping me.

Nancy flew home to Portland this morning, and now I'm alone in my Monterey apartment. The squawk of a seagull echoes down the chimney into the fireplace, interrupting the ghostly quiet. I rearrange the knickknacks on the shelves in the living room, launder the leopard-print sheets from the king-size bed where we both slept, and finish unpacking my suitcases. Nancy was my last connection to the world I've known. During our trip to California—across the plains, through the desert, up the foothills, over the Rockies, and down the east coast of San Francisco Bay—she was my touchstone to the familiar. As the distance stretched farther and farther from my base, she remained a constant. Now she's gone; that final thread is severed. The sun sinks into the Pacific Ocean, and I eat leftovers from last night's dinner at a seafood place.

It seems surreal that I'm in California, that snow-packed Michigan is three time zones away and I don't reside there anymore, at least not for the next six months. I consider the places I've lived—North Dakota, Nebraska, Texas, Nevada, Alaska, California, Minnesota, Michigan—and suddenly realize I've never lived alone before. Never. I've always been surrounded by family or, during my student days, by one or more roommates; have always had someone to talk to, someone to hear my gripes, my pleasures, my worries. I haven't ever been lonely at home. Tonight I miss my husband, my friends, my house, Jim's dog, Joe's cat, the people at work.

I love being here in Monterey, love the lush gardens, the gold rush–era buildings, the breezy California attitude, the lazy harbor seals and raucous sea lions, the waves off the bay that crash against the rocks, the coastal trail where I walk to work every morning and back home every evening. These details decorate the deeper meaning of my being here—my freedom. It's as if I stepped out of one universe—my world in Ann Arbor that is loaded with responsibilities, deadlines, interruptions, sick people—and into the very different world of Monterey—a fairytale place of flowers in winter. I still have responsibilities and deadlines and interruptions, but they don't seem as compelling or overwhelming or oppressive as those at home.

It's ten o'clock in the morning, and I've just finished answering my e-mails from the university in Michigan. I have completed administrative forms, given guidance for the training grant renewal my colleagues are putting together, answered questions from my lab crew, written a letter of recommendation, and reviewed a draft of a scientific manuscript. The three-hour time difference between the East and West Coasts means the workday in Ann Arbor has had a strong start by the time I log on in Monterey.

Time for coffee. Out the backdoor of my MIIS office building, camellias bloom in the alley beside a clump of holly. The florist next door uses this space as overflow storage for his buckets of fresh-cut flowers. I've never seen alleys like this, clean, colorful, full of greenery, full of blossoms. On the way to Morgan's coffee shop, I purchase stamps from the post office, withdraw a hundred dollars from my bank's ATM, deposit two rolls of exposed film at Green's Camera Shop, and buy a tube of toothpaste at the drugstore. In Ann Arbor, running these routine errands is complicated; each consumes time; each requires a trip in the car. Here I can walk all over Old Monterey and, most important, am eager to do that.

At Morgan's I order my usual—double mocha with low-fat milk and no whipped cream—and buy the morning's *New York Times*. This coffee shop is a favorite of Monterey natives. They leisurely sit around the outdoor tables, talking, laughing, reading, eating, just like Ann Arborites do at the coffee shops back home. The difference is that I'm among them here in California; in Ann Arbor I never am.

Outside, the air is clear, cooled by the bay, and the sun, hanging bright in the sky, warms my face. I take a seat on a park bench beside Morgan's, open the newspaper, and sip my drink.

Forty-five minutes later I return, guilt free, to the institute to work on my research project.

In the evenings I read. I write. I listen to NPR and knit. I walk along the coastal trail toward Pacific Grove, in the opposite direction from my route to work, breathing the sea air, the mist from the spindrift, and the ever so faint smell from the California poppies and ice plants. After dark, I gaze out my living room window that overlooks the water, at the lights from the squid boats that make the bay look like a field of night baseball games. In spite of the aloneness, I am exhilarated by my independence. I answer to no one. As my friend Carol says, "You can drink a couple beers for breakfast and don't need to explain it to anybody."

On many weekends, Ray, the director of the Chemical and Biological Weapons Nonproliferation Program at MIIS, leads field trips for the graduate students and junior analysts. He invites me along. Under Ray's command, we hike the grassy slopes of Toro Park on the old Fort Ord Army Base. We crawl through caves and climb the steep, rocky trails at the Pinnacles National Monument. We picnic at the Chalone vineyard. We walk among elephant seals during their annual beaching at the Ano Nuevo State Park. We watch birds at the Moss Landing State Sanctuary. We photograph each other frolicking in the lupine in the foothills of the Gabilan Mountains. We lunch at Ray's favorite haunts across Monterey and Santa Cruz counties. We attend a Celtic folk music festival.

This is all so exciting to me. New people. New places. New sights. New activities. It's exactly the adventure I sought in arranging this sabbatical.

"Would you be willing to give a talk at the biosecurity conference in Almaty, in May?" Ray asks. He leans into my MIIS office, the tiny room with a large window that faces the yellow brick wall three feet away.

Almaty. That's the city in Kazakhstan where MIIS has a small field office.

"Absolutely," I tell Ray. "What do you want me to talk about?" I don't know much about biodefense and less about biosecurity.

"How about scientific ethics and the threat of bioterrorism?"

It's a deal. I know about ethics, at least I understand the moral codes that govern scientific inquiry. In truth, I'd give a lecture on anything to get to go to Kazakhstan.

I'm not sure where that country is, other than it's one of the "Stans" that were once part of the former Soviet Union. I consult the map of the world that hangs on the wall outside my office. There, to the right of the Caspian Sea, below Russia, to the left of China, sits Kazakhstan.

⚘

It's been three days since I arrived in Almaty. Sonya, from the Washington MIIS office, fluent in Russian and a frequent visitor to Kazakhstan, ushers me to a restaurant via the local taxi system. She stands in the street, hails a passing family car, and negotiates the price of a ride.

There's a lull in the music, and it's time to order. We stare at the menus, numbed by the Cyrillic script. Sonya orders for all of us.

"What do you like?" she asks.

"Anything." "Everything," we answer.

"Are you sure?"

Yeah, we're sure. We'll eat whatever the Kazakhs eat.

Soon platters of *manty* (meat dumplings), *lagman* (beef stew over noodles), *plov* (rice pilaf), *kazy* (horsemeat sausage), *besbaramak* (lamb, sour milk, and noodles), and *baursaks* (savory doughnuts) crowd the table before us. Food for nine costs 6,000 *tenge* (US$37.50).

Rich sensations—visual, gustatory, auditory, tactile—throb against us from every corner of this restaurant: the exotic smells and tastes of cooked lamb and onions; the flash of the spotlights reflected off the dancers' bangles and belt buckles; the haunting sounds of the Kazakh singers accompanied by two-stringed dombras that look like small guitars but sound like violins as they beautifully, eerily stir every possible emotion.

My new friends crowd around the dinner table, eating, drinking, laughing, singing. Marina and Aigerim work at the Almaty MIIS office, and Marina's mother, Elena, who speaks no English, has been my personal tour guide. Ray, Rich, and Michael came with me from

MIIS in Monterey. Roger and John are from a peace institute in Sweden. Almaty is a very faraway place, halfway around the world from North Dakota where I grew up. If my girlhood friend Mary Euren and I had been successful when we dug a "hole to China" in her backyard—we gave up at seventeen inches into the dirt—we actually would have ended up in Kazakhstan.

I'm caught in a whirlwind of adventures, visits to the Children's Clinical Hospital and to the Anti-plague Institute in Almaty, vodka-soaked dinners with scientists and government officials throughout the newly independent Central Asian countries. I buy crafts from the artisans' market, dance with the health minister from Tajikistan, lunch beside the wishing tree at Kok-Tubee. For eight nights I sleep in the Russian-era Dostyk Hotel with screenless windows that open to admit the fresh spring air. None of it would have happened without my cancer. It took a malignancy to get me here.

Before leaving California for the drive back to Michigan with Jim, I buy a redwood tree seedling. Planted in a clay pot, it basks in the daylight from my living room window that overlooks Monterey Bay. Hopefully it will survive the road trip to Ann Arbor. This little tree will be a constant reminder of my unhampered freedom while in Monterey. Like an adopted child, it will grow up in a new place.

Michigan, of course, has seasons: hot, humid summers; frigid, dry winters; glorious springs; bracing falls. My little tree's DNA isn't programmed to cope with the seasons. But, I'll keep it indoors, where it's always seventy-two degrees. I'm certain it will thrive there.

# CHAPTER 20

Restructuring a Life

*The Squaw Valley Community of Writers* (SVCW) is sponsoring a new conference entitled "Writing the Medical Experience." Although I've attended many summer writing workshops—in Minnesota, Cape Cod, Maine—none have focused solely on a literary medical theme. To apply to the program, I send a draft of a short story I've written about the boardroom fantasies of a corporate woman with a mutilated breast following cancer surgery. Wonder where that came from.

Admission to SVCW is highly competitive, and I'm honored, and a bit surprised, to be accepted. In the shadow of California's Sierra Nevada mountains, we gather—physicians, nurses, social workers, and patients who are also poets, novelists, short fiction writers, and essayists.

I've been assigned a bedroom in a condo on the valley floor. The view from the living room window is breathtaking: rock outcroppings jut between the pines, the dull, blue-gray granite plays against the clear azure sky. The view of the basin, however, is tragic. The creek, which once wound leisurely through a meadow of wild flowers, has been rerouted into a straight line and now races through an absurdly lush golf course.

The condo's other bedroom has two beds, and I'm expecting roommates. As I unpack my suitcase, they arrive.

"Hi," the younger woman says in a lightly Irish brogue as she bounces through the door. "I'm Shannon and this is my mother, Mary."

We finish the introductions—where we live, how we learned of this workshop, why we chose to attend, what we are writing.

"Shannon and I have just finished a book about our experiences with breast cancer," Mary says in her rolling, southern drawl.

I look from one to the other, from the daughter born in Ireland to the mother born in Tennessee. "You both had breast cancer?"

"Yes," they answer, nodding, in unison.

"Well, so did I."

In the early mornings, we chat about our cancers. Mid-mornings we walk through the village to our workshops. Afternoons we attend lectures, and early evenings we attend readings. Later, into the night, Mary, Shannon, and I talk again. Their family has a tragic, four-generation history of breast cancer, and we contemplate the meaning of this legacy for their daughters. Shannon is healthy after a bilateral mastectomy, and Mary has metastatic disease.

"See," she says, opening her shirt. The skin over her clavicle is pocked with cancerous lumps.

We talk about operations, about chemo, about Mary's implant gone awry, about Shannon's decision against reconstruction, about our disease.

"As soon as I get back home, I start more chemo," Mary says, running her fingers through her honey hair. "I guess it'll all fall out again. That'll be the third time."

When Shannon is out of earshot, Mary asks about squirreling away drugs so she can control her future when it becomes no longer bearable. "Which pills should I hoard?" "How many would I need?"

I suggest she get that information from the Hemlock Society in the library or on the Web. "But, Mary," I say, "keep all your options open. I strongly suggest you look into hospice when you get home. It may not be for you, but at least learn what they can offer."

The next day, the three of us are walking across the courtyard when Mary suddenly falls to the pavement. My heart lurches into my throat. It's a brain met, I think to myself, and she's had a stroke. Or a pathologic fracture from a metastasis in her hip bone.

"Just stumbled." She tries to get up. "I'll be fine."

We help her stand, but she can't walk on her left foot, so Shannon suggests going back to the condo.

"No." Mary is resolute. "I'm not missing this afternoon's session." She insists on returning to her classroom. With one hand on the stair rail and the other on me, Mary hops, one-footed, up the narrow flight of steps.

In the afternoon, Shannon drives her mother to an orthopedic surgeon in town, who diagnoses a sprained ankle. Later Mary hobbles into the apartment on crutches, her leg secured in a brace. "It's always something," she says. At least this time it isn't cancer.

We read each other's literary work. Their book is beautiful. The naked honesty of their words is stunning. No sugarcoating for these two.

Mary's chapters begin with poems.

"You're a poet?" I ask.

"Never thought I was," Mary grins. "I wrote what came into my head, and when I showed it to a friend, she said it was poetry. 'Baloney!' I said. But when she rearranged the words on the page, they turned into poems."

Mary complains about the lymphedema in her arm. She's been bundling it in layers of stockinette, foam, and Ace wraps, which she can't get on straight. I show her how to apply them correctly.

"Jan . . . et," she calls from their room at bedtime, "could you help tie me up?" She doesn't like wearing the wraps during the day because they're so hot and bulky. I give her one of my elastic pressure sleeves, but it's too big and hangs from her arm like a pajama top. My compression glove, though, fits, so she wears it the rest of the week.

The night before we leave, Mary complains of a swollen eye. "Damn allergies," she mumbles, limping out of their bedroom. "Do you have any antihistamines?"

"Let me see." I examine her eye. I'm not at all sure this is allergies. "I have Sudafed but no antihistamines. As soon as you get back to Washington, you'd better check this out with your doctor."

Mary is silent.

"Promise?"

"OK, I will," she mutters.

The next day we say good-bye to each other, to our writing classmates, and depart, promising to stay in touch.

Now that I'm home from Monterey, all the stuff around my house irritates me. I lived for six months in California with only my belongings that fit into the PT Cruiser, and I lived very well. So much of the detritus that surrounds me here is outdated, out of style, redundant. I need to streamline, lighten the load, free myself from the weight of all this junk.

So I purge. Every closet, cabinet, and drawer in the house is scrutinized. I'm ruthless. If it hasn't been worn in three years, it goes to the Purple Heart Charities. Piles of catalogs, my twenty-year stash of wine bottle corks, books I'll never open again, leftover yarn I wouldn't be able to knit up even if I live to be 130. Recipes for dishes I will never cook. Jewelry. Cosmetics, including those left over from the "Look Good, Feel Better" program. Two decades of dry-cleaner hangers. Twin bed sheets—there hasn't been a twin-size bed in this house for over ten years. These possessions are moldering, unused, taking up space. For me they no longer represent security against an unexpected crisis, as in "you never know when you'll need three fondue pots." Maybe perceived crises don't drive my actions much anymore, or maybe I don't perceive the issues as crises. Whatever, this stuff is like an anchor tied to my waist and stuck in the muddy bottom of a lake. In the unlikely event I discover a need for more than one fondue pot, I'll buy a new one.

When I finally finish cleaning out, I survey my home. It's sleeker, more spacious, more functional. The air circulates more freely. I'm more comfortable here. This space fits me better now.

The Cancer Center examination rooms look a lot like the rooms in the pediatric clinic. The tools I use for my work hang on the wall here, too: ophthalmoscope, otoscope, ear specula in three sizes, blood pressure cuff and sphygmomanometer. Beside the sink hangs a framed print of three floating lily pads. In my clinic rooms, however, there are no pictures. Rather, toys are mounted on the walls so that the children can spin colorful plastic gears or make shadowy palm prints—or, as enterprising boys sometimes do, sole-of-the-foot prints.

Here I'm still the patient, still wear the hospital gown backwards.

"How are you doing?" my oncologist asks.

"I am great," I answer and point to the patient history forms where I have circled

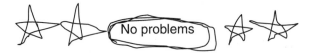

After my visit with my doctor I ask the checkout clerk, a young man with a broad smile, "Are you open for business?"

"Sure," he answers, reaching for my papers. "Will you need a follow-up appointment?"

"In six months."

This visit has gone without a hitch. What happened? Have I changed, or have they?

* * *

There's a rainbow arching over Geddes Road. Red, orange, yellow, green, blue, indigo, violet—the colors melt into each other. As I drive toward it, one end seems to drop into a pot of gold buried on the exit ramp from northbound U.S. 23. How many rainbows have I seen in my life? Hundreds. Why do I particularly note this one? Because its colors are more vibrant than any of those other rainbows? Because the payoff is within reach? How many more rainbows will I see?

A ratty tennis shoe languishes beside Huron Parkway, among the weeds, in the rain, without its mate. Why does the sight of this lost shoe make me so sad this afternoon?

The Gewandhaus Orchestra of Leipzig fills the stage of Hill Auditorium. From our seats in the second row of the lower balcony, Sally and I listen to Beethoven's Fourth Symphony. I aim my opera glasses at one of the flutists. The part in her straight brown hair, which is pulled behind her ears, is a little off center. She wears a simple black dress with caped shoulders and no makeup. Her face is solemn, unsmiling.

But her music is glorious. The notes are light-footed and as lyrical as a lullaby. She moves as she plays, raising her elbows as the tones raise, swaying forward to coax more sound from her instrument, swooping her body to the rhythm of the second movement.

How many Beethoven symphonies have I heard in my life? The flutist and her music make this performance more vibrant than I can ever remember. How many more Beethoven symphonies will I hear again? How many more concerts in Hill Auditorium?

Jim makes an ill-advised investment and loses some of our retirement fund. He's reluctant to tell me, afraid "The Wrath of Janet" will fall upon him. When I get the news, I shake my head and shrug, "It's only money."

An e-mail arrives from a medical friend whose wife has just been diagnosed with breast cancer. He's terrified, convinced he has lost the partner he has loved for so long. He asks what life is like, now that I have completed therapy.

> From: Janet Gilsdorf
> To: rvivuv@yahoo.com
> Date: August 28, 2002 4:03:42 PM
> Subject: Re: greetings
> Rob,
> Great to hear from you. I've been thinking about
> you and Elaine a lot. I'm pleased to hear she's
> doing so well. Your strength of character will get
> you both through this.
> To answer your question in a roundabout way . . .
> When I was undergoing treatment, Claire asked the
> key question—"What proportion of your waking hours
> are you aware that you have cancer?" My answer then
> was about 85%. My answer today would be <1% and

only when triggered by outside reminders. When my
left arm feels as if it's immersed in ice water or
when I tug at my compression sleeve to make it fit
better, I don't think "cancer." If I think at all,
I think "troublesome arm."
It's interesting to consider how my breast cancer
has become just another, albeit important, chapter
in my book of life.
I'm in awe of the many ways my illness has liber-
ated me. I doubt I would have had the gumption to
go off on my own to Monterey and to Kazakhstan
without it. I certainly enjoy a broader relationship with the world and have a lot more material to
write about!!!!
Please stay in touch.
Janet

After hitting the "send" button, I sit back and think about what
I've told him. I said I am consciously aware of having cancer less than
1 percent of the time. Is that right? How about deeper than conscious-
ness? How about at the bottom of the farthest reach of my psyche?

Do I obsess about cancer? No. Do I walk around in a state of panic
that I'm going to find a metastasis next week, that I'm going to die of
my cancer? No. Does it live with me, always, and tint my worldview?
Yes.

The memo that I sent to Rob was the public face of my cancer.
There is a private face to it, one that I hear in the music of my new *All
Songs Considered* CD from NPR; that I see in the faces of my patients
as they struggle to conquer their illnesses and of my students as they
learn medicine and infectious diseases; that I hear in the telephone
voices of my sons from faraway places; that I read in the written words
of Michael Ondaatje and Anne Lamott and Ann Patchett.

Like a shadow, it follows me to San Juan Island in Puget Sound, to
Puerto de Santa Maria in Spain. It's with me in my chair as I read the
*New York Times* and as I drive Plymouth Road to work.

If my life were a book, what would be the section topics? What are
the events that made a permanent stamp on who I am?

1. Infancy in Minneapolis
2. Growing up in Fargo, North Dakota
3. Attending medical school
4. Marrying Jim
5. Living on an Indian reservation in Nevada and in the middle of the tundra in Alaska
6. Mothering Dan and Joe
7. Being a university faculty member
8. Having cancer
9.

How about number 9? And 19?

Shannon sends me an e-mail. "That swollen eye wasn't allergies," she writes. "It was a metastasis in Mum's brain."

As I stare at her words on my computer's screen, a breath-stopping ache claws through me. I think of Mary and her vitality, her soaring spirit, her creativity. She struck me as the current Mother Superior in a dynasty of able women. The tragedy of Mary's dynasty is that it's infected with a very bad gene.

Shannon writes often. Her mother is in a great deal of pain. The hospice nurse isn't doing her job. I'm livid and urge Shannon to tell the oncologist, tell the agency. She does, and Mary's pain comes under control.

A week later, Mary is no longer responsive. She's cloistered in her private, hopefully peaceful, world.

Six weeks after we left Squaw Valley, Mary is dead. She remains with me like an echo—a treasured, golden echo. We spent one short week together, but her influence is boundless. Now she's gone. . . .

The voices irritate me. On this sunny summer morning seated on my back porch amid the geraniums and petunias, I'm trying to write, and the noise distracts me. Even worse is the honking car horns. And the yelling.

I give up on writing at home and decide to go to the office. As I change into my professional clothes, I remember the signs along the street and the radio announcements and realize what the racket is all about. It's a walkathon to earn money for the Susan G. Komen Foundation. It's one of those pink ribbon, cancer sorority fund-raising events, and it's snaking down Plymouth Road, not two hundred yards from my porch.

I drive out of my neighborhood and pass phalanxes of the marathon walkers. Most are women. A few are men. Old, young, fat, skinny, black, white. Hundreds and hundreds wearing walking shoes and identical T-shirts. Some tote day packs, some sport head rags, some carry water bottles that dangle from their belts. I can't read the words on the shirts. To get a closer look, I pull into the street beside the Old Dixboro School, where the playground is littered with canopies, tents, tables of rehydration jugs, rows of Porta Potties. From here I can read the logo on the fronts of the walkers: "Breast Cancer 3•Day."

These people are walking sixty miles to earn money for breast cancer. One woman uses a cane. Another limps on an ankle brace. They won't make it to the end, not the whole sixty miles. But they are doing what they can.

Suddenly, a flood of emotion washes over me. I rest my forehead on the steering wheel. An intimacy between these walkers and my disease pounds at me. The folks in this marathon are taking this trek because they believe they can make a difference, because they want to honor women who have suffered the ravages of breast cancer. Women like Mary. Like Shannon. Like me.

When my tears clear so I can see, I turn the car around and return home. I want to write again, want to capture this moment. The noise is no longer a distraction. It's more like an affirmation.

On a blank screen of my computer I type:

*Long. Hard. Illuminating. Sometimes full, sometimes empty. Laced with improbable beauty. This was my journey.*

Text design by Mary H. Sexton

Typesetting by Delmastype, Ann Arbor, Michigan

Text Font: Fournier MT

In 1924, Monotype based this face on types cut by Pierre Simon
Fournier circa 1742. These types were some of the most influential
designs of the eighteenth century, being among the earliest of the
"transitional" style of typeface, and were a stepping stone to the more
severe "modern" style made popular by Bodoni later in the century.
Fournier has a light, clean look on the page, provides good economy
in text and retains an even color.

—Courtesy www.adobe.com

Ornament Font: Golden Cockerel

In 1928–29 Eric Gill, designer of Gill Sans and Perpetua, was com-
missioned to produce a typeface for the Golden Cockerel a private
English press press. Digital revivals of the Golden Cockerel type
were made by ITC in 1995–96.

—Courtesy www.myfonts.com

CONVERSATIONS IN MEDICINE AND SOCIETY

THE CONVERSATIONS IN MEDICINE AND SOCIETY series
publishes innovative, accessible, and provocative books on a range of
topics related to health, society, culture, and policy in modern America
(1900 to the present). Current and upcoming titles focus on the historical,
social, and cultural dimensions of health and sickness, public policy,
medical professionalization, and subjective experiences of illness.

SERIES EDITORS
Howard Markel and Alexandra Minna Stern,
University of Michigan

*Formative Years: Children's Health in the United States, 1800–2000*
edited by Alexandra Minna Stern and Howard Markel

*The DNA Mystique: The Gene as Cultural Icon*
by Dorothy Nelkin and M. Susan Lindee

*Universal Coverage: The Elusive Quest for National Health Insurance*
by Rick Mayes

*The Midnight Meal and Other Essays About Doctors, Patients, and Medicine*
by Jerome Lowenstein

*Deadly Dust: Silicosis and the On-Going Struggle to Protect Workers' Health*
by David Rosner and Gerald Markowitz

*Inside/Outside: A Physician's Journey with Cancer*
by Janet R. Gilsdorf